Food for Health

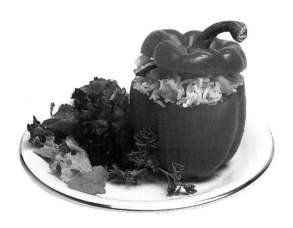

Dr John Briffa

BSc (Hons) MB BS (Lond)

MARSHALL PUBLISHING • LONDON

A Marshall Edition
Conceived, edited and designed by
Marshall Editions
161 New Bond Street, London W1Y 9PA

First published in the UK in 1998 by
Marshall Publishing Ltd

ISBN: 1 84028 145 6

Originated in the UK by DP Graphics
Printed and bound in Portugal by
Printer Portuguesa

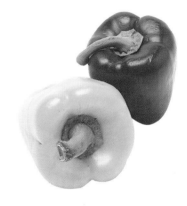

Project Editor Cathy Meeus

Art Editor Hugh Schermuly

Designer Sally Geeve

Copy Editor Anna Selby

Food Stylist Jacqueline Bellefontaine

Indexer Lynn Bresler

Picture Research Zilda Tandy

Managing Editor Anne Yelland

Editorial Director Sophie Collins

Art Director Sean Keogh

Editorial Coordinator Becca Clunes

Production Nikki Ingram

Note

Every effort has been taken to ensure that all information in this book is correct and compatible with national standards generally accepted at the time of publication. This book is not intended to replace consultation with your doctor or other healthcare professional. The author and publisher disclaim any liability, loss, injury or damage incurred as a consequence, directly or indirectly, of the use and application of the contents of this book.

CONTENTS

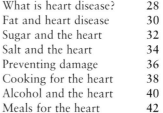

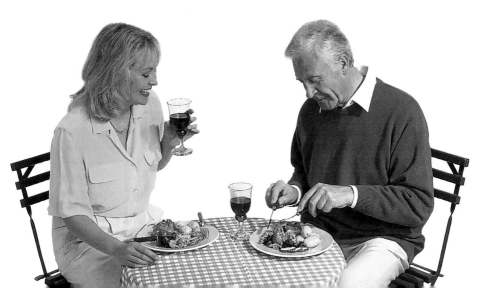

Eating for Digestive Health

Eating for Weight Control

Eating for Immune Health

Shopping and Cooking

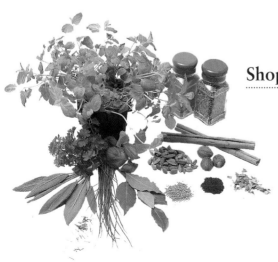

INTRODUCTION

Good health is our most valuable commodity. Feeling fit and well, both physically and mentally, is a natural and instinctive part of everyday life. However, we rarely appreciate the true value of good health until we fall ill. In other words, most of us take our health for granted.

WHAT DETERMINES GOOD HEALTH?

Many factors affect our health and wellbeing. The important influences are; genetics, our environment, the type of health care we receive, and our lifestyle. It is easy to overestimate the impact on our health of some of these factors. For example, it has been estimated that conventional medical treatment contributes only about 10 per cent to our overall health, while genetic factors probably account for around another 20 per cent.

THE IMPACT OF LIFESTYLE

The most significant statistic is, however, that aspects of lifestyle account for about 50 per cent of the factors that determine health. What this means is that disease is rarely solely the result of some unlucky whim of fate or genetics, it is more often the result of how we choose to live our lives. Of the lifestyle factors, diet plays a central role. There is a growing body of evidence that shows just how important our food choices are in enhancing health, preventing illness and prolonging life. This book has been written to give you a clear understanding of how food affects all aspects of your health.

RENEWAL AND REPAIR

The human body is constantly renewing itself. Every moment of every day the body's basic constituents are wearing out, only to be replaced with new tissues and biochemical components. About 98 per cent of the body is completely remade this way each year. The raw materials

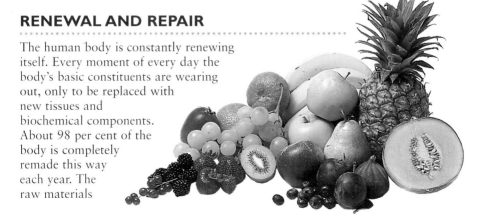

that your body uses to rebuild itself come almostly exclusively from from food. What this means is that your body is essentially composed of what you have eaten over the last year. From this perspective it is easy to appreciete the impact that diet has on our health and welbeing.

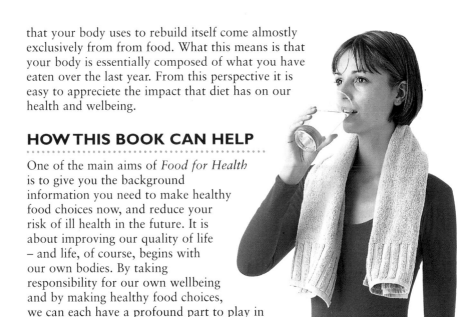

HOW THIS BOOK CAN HELP

One of the main aims of *Food for Health* is to give you the background information you need to make healthy food choices now, and reduce your risk of ill health in the future. It is about improving our quality of life – and life, of course, begins with our own bodies. By taking responsibility for our own wellbeing and by making healthy food choices, we can each have a profound part to play in our future health and happiness.

HOW TO USE THIS BOOK

This book is divided into six chapters, each of which deals with a different body function and how it contributes to health and wellbeing – energy, the heart, the digestive system, weight control and the immune system. Each chapter explains the impact of diet on that particular system – including those foods that enhance health and those that may harm it. The final chapter deals with the all-important area of food shopping and preparation. There is also a final section devoted to menu plans to provide practical help in making healthy changes in your eating habits. If you know which subject area you wish to access, turn to the relevant tab. On each you will find a detailed table of contents of that section of the guide. If you are unsure where to find the information you need, turn to the alphabetical index on page 112.

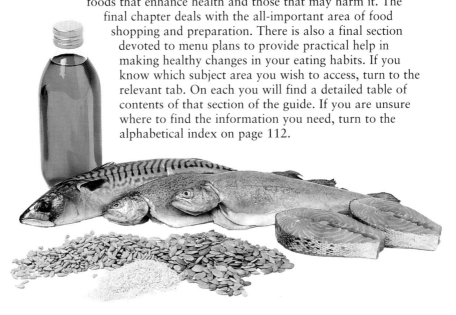

EATING FOR ENERGY

Lack of energy and vitality is perhaps the most common of everyday complaints. Many people find that each day brings periods of near exhaustion. This low level of energy may, in fact, be closely related to diet. By choosing the best fuel for the body, you can promote dramatic improvements in energy levels and a generally enhanced sense of well being. Whether you suffer from low blood sugar, want to improve your energy level for sport or keep your bones strong and healthy as you get older, eating a good diet can help.

GENERATING ENERGY

The food we eat is the raw fuel our bodies use to generate energy. Just as a fire needs logs or coal to keep it burning, so we, too, need food to keep the body working properly. However, getting energy from our diet is a complex process and not simply a matter of putting the right food in our mouths.

FROM FOOD TO ENERGY

The release of energy from food is dependent on four essential steps:

1 Digestion After food has been swallowed, it passes into the digestive tract. Food is progressively broken down by chewing and the effects of acid in the stomach and of digestive enzymes in the small intestine so that the nutrients can be absorbed through the gut wall into the bloodstream.

2 Food processing Food molecules that have been absorbed from the gut into the bloodstream initially pass to the liver. Some food particles are broken down still further here, while others are converted into forms that can be used to store fuel around the body.

3 Transport When the food has been processed by the liver, it is dissolved in the bloodstream to be transported to wherever it is needed in the body.

4 Metabolism Metabolism is the process by which food is "burnt" with oxygen to create energy and it actually takes place within the body's basic building blocks – the cells. The body is made up of trillions of cells, each of which has the capacity to absorb food molecules, subjecting them to chemical reactions which generate energy. To function efficiently, these reactions require a range of nutrients.

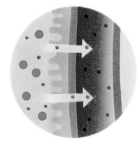 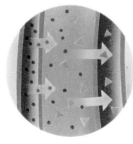 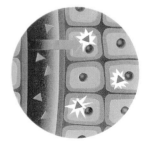

Food is broken down into small particles by the processes of digestion in the mouth, stomach and small intestine.

The food particles are small enough to pass through the wall of the small intestine into the bloodstream.

Having been further processed in the liver, nutrients from food can pass into the cells where they can be used to create energy or to build new cells.

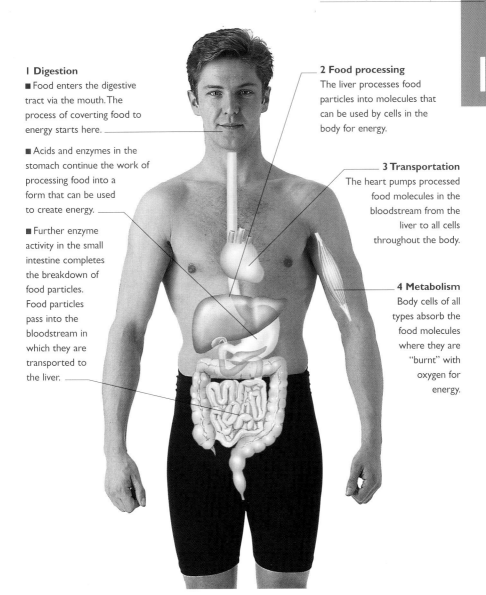

I Digestion

■ Food enters the digestive tract via the mouth. The process of coverting food to energy starts here.

■ Acids and enzymes in the stomach continue the work of processing food into a form that can be used to create energy.

■ Further enzyme activity in the small intestine completes the breakdown of food particles. Food particles pass into the bloodstream in which they are transported to the liver.

2 Food processing
The liver processes food particles into molecules that can be used by cells in the body for energy.

3 Transportation
The heart pumps processed food molecules in the bloodstream from the liver to all cells throughout the body.

4 Metabolism
Body cells of all types absorb the food molecules where they are "burnt" with oxygen for energy.

WHEN THE PROCESS FAILS

If any of these essential processes falters, energy production in the body may stall. For instance, poor digestion can lead to inadequate absorption of nutrients from the intestine which in turn will starve the body of fuel. One or more nutritional deficiencies can also lead to an inefficiency in the reactions that generate energy within the cell. Keeping our energy-producing systems in good working order really depends on healthy digestive, circulatory and biochemical functions within the body.

ENERGY STORES

Fuel in the body is stored in three main forms. The most readily available fuel source in the body is sugar in the bloodstream. While this can be used to generate energy very quickly, it is in limited supply. Blood sugar levels must therefore be continually topped up from a bigger store of fuel. This larger fuel store is provided by a substance called glycogen which is similar in structure to starch. Glycogen is stored in the muscles and the liver and is quite readily converted into sugar which can then be burnt for energy. The third energy store in the body is fat. Much more energy can be stored as fat in the body than as glycogen, but the body finds it harder to convert this form of fuel into energy for instant use.

THE ENERGY BANK

To use money as an analogy for the body's energy stores, sugar in the bloodstream would be the money in our pocket or purse – easy to get hold of but in relatively short supply; glycogen would be a current account in the bank, that can keep the money in our purse or pocket topped up; finally, fat would be the deposit account, where the bulk of our money is kept but to which access is more limited.

ENERGY STORES

Energy for the body

Blood sugar

Sugar in the bloodstream is used for immediate energy.

Glycogen

Glycogen in the muscles and liver is used as an energy source when blood sugar is used up.

Fat

Energy stored in the form of fat is the body's last resort for its energy supply and is not easily "accessed".

ENERGY-GIVING FOOD

The three main energy-giving constituents of the food we eat are carbohydrate, fat and protein. It is the relative proportions of these basic elements that makes a particular food a good or poor source of energy for the body.

CARBOHYDRATE

Carbohydrates come in the form of sugars and starches. The basic unit of a carbohydrate is the monosaccharide molecule, the most common form of which is glucose (a sugar). Starch is actually composed of long chains of individual monosaccharide molecules. The amount of energy that foods release when they are metabolized in the body's cells is measured in calories. Carbohydrates give up about 4 kilocalories of energy for each gram that is burnt. The body has only a limited ability to produce sugar in the bloodstream from substances other than carbohydrates. This means that consuming a diet high in carbohydrates is essential for energy. High carbohydrate foods include bread, rice, pasta, crackers, breakfast cereals, potatoes, dried fruit, fruit, beans, pulses, jam and honey.

FAT

Fat's basic component is the triglyceride molecule. Triglyceride molecules are broken down by digestion prior to absorption into the bloodstream. Some of their basic components are burnt as fuel, liberating about 9 kilocalories of energy for each gram of fat that is burnt. However, most of the triglycerides that come from the diet are reconstituted back into fat for storage in the body. While high-fat foods can help replenish fuel stores in the body, they do not provide a ready source of energy and may also have harmful effects on health if eaten in excess. High-fat foods include butter, margarine, oils, meat (especially beef, lamb, pork and duck), sausages, pâté and cheese.

PROTEIN

Proteins are large molecules which, when broken down, yield single units called amino acids. Amino acids are primarily required in the body for the structural components of many tissues such as muscle, hormones and digestive enzymes. Under extreme conditions, such as starvation and when relatively little energy can be derived from depleted fat and carbohydrate reserves, amino acids may be used to provide energy. Protein liberates about 4 kilocalories of energy for each gram of protein that is burnt. However, in general daily life, only a very small amount of energy comes from protein in the diet. High-protein foods include meat, offal, fish, milk, cheese, yoghurt and eggs.

BLOOD SUGAR

Fuel in the body is stored as fat and as the starch-like substance, glycogen (see page 10). However, for us to be able to generate energy, fuel stores must first be converted into sugar. Sugar in the bloodstream is the essential accessible fuel in the body. However full the body's fat and glycogen stores may be, if there is not enough sugar in the blood-stream, the body will be unable to make adequate amounts of energy.

FROM CARBOHYDRATE TO ENERGY

Carbohydrate is the main source of energy in the diet, but it must undergo a series of processes before it is available to the body. When a carbohydrate is eaten, it is broken down into simple sugars by digestive enzymes which can then pass through the gut wall into the bloodstream. As these molecules are absorbed, the blood sugar level starts to rise. The pancreas, a tapered organ that lies behind the stomach, responds to rising levels of sugar in the bloodstream by secreting a hormone called insulin. This essential hormone facilitates the absorption of sugar into the body's cells. The action of insulin, which makes sugars available for energy production, is also essential to the regulation of healthy blood sugar levels.

Warning!

While symptoms of low energy may often be related to low blood sugar, medical conditions such as diabetes (below), anaemia and low thyroid function may also have fatigue as a major symptom. Always consult your doctor if you are suffering from persistent tiredness.

DIABETES

Diabetes mellitus or "sugar diabetes" is now the third leading cause of death in the western world. Although diabetics often lead apparently active, normal lives, diabetes is a serious condition with debilitating complications that may reduce overall life expectancy by about a third.

Diabetes mellitus is a condition in which sugar metabolism is disordered and blood sugar levels tend to be higher than desired. Type II or adult-onset diabetes accounts for the 90 per cent of diabetes cases that commence in middle or old age when the body seems to develop a resistance to the effects of insulin. Type II diabetics can normally control their condition with dietary modifications and/or oral medication and so the term non-insulin dependent diabetes is also used to describe this condition. However, insulin is sometimes used if these measures prove inadequate.

The dietary guidelines for a non-insulin dependent diabetic are the same as those for an individual suffering from hypoglycaemia. Meals should be taken on a regular basis and the diet should be based on low glycaemic index foods (see page 15).

WHAT IS LOW BLOOD SUGAR?

Many people who complain of unexplained tiredness tend to have a lower than normal level of sugar in the bloodstream. Low blood sugar – also known as hypoglycaemia – causes tiredness because without sugar the body cannot generate energy. Low blood sugar can occur even in those who have long-term energy stores in the form of glycogen or body fat, but who for some reason cannot convert these stores to sugar for use as energy. It is a bit like having a blockage in the fuel line to the engine of a car. The tank may be full but the car still won't start. There are a number of possible causes of low blood sugar. It is normal for blood sugar to become depleted if you miss a meal or if you have expended a lot of energy without additional food intake. Some people have an inborn tendency to the problem. Most types of low blood sugar can be avoided by eating the right kinds of food and by keeping to regular mealtimes.

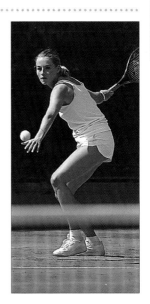

COMMON SYMPTOMS OF LOW BLOOD SUGAR

■ **Fluctuating energy with fatigue being worst on waking and in the middle to the late afternoon** Energy can be low in the morning despite adequate sleep because the blood sugar level tends to fall overnight. Low blood sugar can occur in the middle or late afternoon because the body can often over-compensate for the increase in blood sugar after lunch, leading to low blood sugar some hours later.

■ **Weakness, light-headedness or irritability if a meal is skipped or delayed** Failing to provide the body with adequate fuel on a regular basis will tend to cause the blood sugar level to drop. Weakness, light-headedness and irritability are symptoms indicative of a brain and body starved of their essential fuel source.

■ **Periodic problems with concentration** The brain uses a large proportion of the sugar in the bloodstream. A lack of sugar supply to the brain will cause problems with mental function, especially concentration. This is a common symptom of low blood sugar in the mid afternoon.

■ **Periodic problems with low mood, depression or irritability** Low sugar supply to the brain can commonly produce changes in mood leading to low mood, depression or irritability.

■ **Food cravings, especially for sweet and/or starchy foods** When blood sugar is low, it is natural for the body to demand foods that release sugar quickly into the bloodstream. Cravings for chocolates, biscuits and other sugary foods are a common feature of low blood sugar.

SUSTAINING BLOOD SUGAR

Eating the right diet is essential in overcoming low blood sugar. People who have a tendency to the problem should eat little and often to ensure that the blood sugar level never gets the opportunity to drop into the danger zone – ideally, allowing no more than three to four hours without eating. The diet should be based on foods that release sugar slowly into the bloodstream.

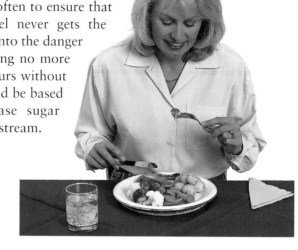

Avoid low blood sugar by eating regular meals that are high in foods that release energy slowly.

MEASURING SUGAR RELEASE

The rate at which foods release sugar into the bloodstream is quantified using a measure called the glycaemic index. Foods that are digested rapidly have a moderate or high glycaemic index (more than 50), while foods that are digested more slowly have a low glycaemic index (less than 50). Sugary and some starchy foods tend to have a high glycaemic index, whereas proteins and vegetables have a low glycaemic index. The ratings of a range of common foods according to the glycaemic index are shown on the facing page.

HOW TO COMBAT LOW BLOOD SUGAR

■ Base your diet around foods of low glycaemic index. This means eating mostly fruit and vegetables, wholegrains, beans, pulses, and some meat and fish.

■ Avoid foods of high glycaemic index because of their tendency to induce low blood sugar some time after their ingestion.

■ If you eat high glycaemic index foods, combine them with foods of lower glycaemic index. A baked potato, for instance, could be eaten with cottage cheese, tuna or chicken and salad or vegetables.

■ Do not skip meals. Eat three meals a day with healthy snacks, such as fruit, in between if necessary.

VERY HIGH GLYCAEMIC INDEX FOODS (OVER 100)

Cornflakes
Glucose
Maltose
Puffed rice
Rice cakes
White bread

HIGH GLYCAEMIC INDEX FOODS (80-100)

Bananas
Brown rice
Carrots
Corn
Corn chips
Mangoes
Muesli
Oat bran
Parsnips

Potatoes
Raisins
Rye crackers
White rice
Wholegrain bread

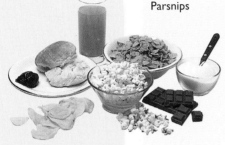

Foods that have a high glycaemic index are generally those that are high in refined carbohydrates and sugar.

MODERATE GLYCAEMIC INDEX FOODS (50-80)

Kidney beans (canned)
Lactose
Oranges
Peas
Potato crisps
Pumpernickel bread
Sucrose
White and wholewheat pasta

LOW GLYCAEMIC INDEX (30-50)

Apples
Barley
Chick peas
Kidney beans (dried)
Lentils
Milk
Peaches
Pears
Wholegrain rye bread
Yoghurt

VERY LOW GLYCAEMIC INDEX FOODS (UNDER 30)

Butter
Cheese
Eggs
Fish

Fructose
Grapefruit
Green vegetables
Meat

Peanuts
Plums
Seafood
Soya beans

NUTRIENTS FOR ENERGY

The primary ingredients that the body uses to generate energy are glucose (sugar) and oxygen. However, the mechanisms that enable the body to convert sugar and oxygen into energy also require a variety of vitamins and minerals. For example, the red blood cells responsible for transporting oxygen around the body depend on certain nutrients for their manufacture. Yet more nutrients are essential for the proper functioning of the muscles.

NUTRIENT	ROLE	SOURCES
Vitamins B$_1$ (thiamin), B$_2$ (riboflavin) and B$_3$ (niacin) 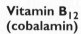	Essential for the reactions that convert food into energy. They are also known to compensate for the effects of stress.	Unrefined wholegrains (brown rice, wholemeal bread, etc), liver, green leafy vegetables, fish, poultry, eggs, red meat, nuts, beans, pulses.
Vitamin B$_5$ (pantothenic acid)	Necessary for the metabolism of carbohydrate, protein and fat. Also needed for red blood cell production.	Eggs; saltwater fish; pork, beef, milk, wholemeal bread, fresh vegetables.
Vitamin B$_{12}$ (cobalamin)	Necessary for the production of red blood cells. Involved in carbohydrate and fat metabolism.	Kidney, liver, egg, herring, mackerel, milk, cheese, tofu, seafood.
Folic acid	Necessary for the production of red blood cells. Involved in protein metabolism.	Beef, lamb, pork, chicken, green leafy vegetables, wholemeal bread, bran.

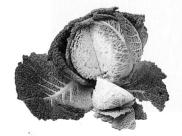

NUTRIENT	ROLE	SOURCES
Iron	Essential for red blood cell formation. Necessary for energy production.	Meat, poultry, eggs, green leafy vegetables, wholemeal bread.
Chromium	Important in glucose metabolism and for maintaining blood sugar stability.	Brewer's yeast, wholegrains, meat, cheese.
Calcium 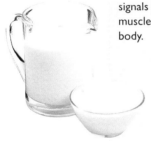	Needed for transmission of nerve signals and proper muscle function in the body.	Milk and milk products, salmon, sardines, seeds, green leafy vegetables, seafood. 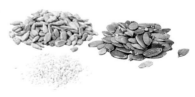
Magnesium	Involved in transmission of nerve signals and necessary for proper muscle function.	Dairy products, meat, fish, green leafy vegetables, seeds.
Potassium	Necessary for nerve transmission and muscle function.	Fresh fruit (especially bananas) and vegetables.

AN ACTIVE LIFESTYLE

Sugar (glucose) in the bloodstream provides the raw fuel necessary for physical activity. During exercise blood sugar levels are topped up from the glycogen stores in the liver and muscles. Anyone taking regular exercise has to maintain a good store of glycogen. This is especially true for those engaged in endurance sports such as running, cycling and rowing. The only way to keep the muscles well stocked with glycogen is to consume adequate amounts of carbohydrates on a regular basis. Starchy foods such as bread, potato, rice and pasta are all high in carbohydrates. However, some carbohydrates are far better than others at providing a sustained source of fuel for the body.

THE GLYCOGEN STORES

If glycogen stores are not adequately topped up between training sessions, the level of glycogen in the body can gradually become depleted over a period of time. If there is only a small amount of fuel in store, it can seriously hamper physical performance. The phenomenon of "hitting the wall", common in marathon runners and other endurance athletes, comes about when glycogen stores in the body have been run down to nothing. The chart below shows how physical activity not adequately balanced by carbohydrate intake can progressively use up stored glycogen, leading to exhaustion. This is compared to an energy-maintaining pattern of glycogen use and replacement, where there is regular replenishment of the glycogen stores.

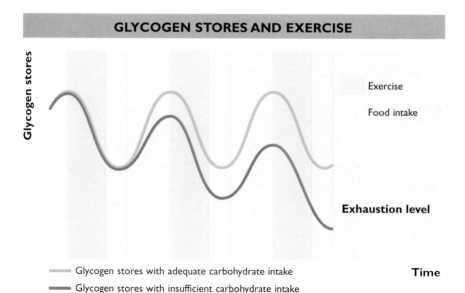

GLYCOGEN STORES AND EXERCISE

Glycogen stores

Exercise

Food intake

Exhaustion level

Time

Glycogen stores with adequate carbohydrate intake

Glycogen stores with insufficient carbohydrate intake

SPORTS DIET

The optimum sports diet should be based on foods that release sugar slowly into the bloodstream such as fresh fruit, vegetables (other than potatoes), and wholegrains such as brown rice, wholewheat pasta, oats and wholemeal bread. These foods release sugar gradually, which is essential for efficient exercise and they are also valuable sources of fibre, vitamins and minerals. Foods that release sugar more quickly, such as potatoes, white rice and non-wholewheat pasta, are best eaten in combination with plenty of salad or vegetables as this tends to buffer the rate at which sugar is released into the bloodstream.

TIMING MEALS

When you eat can be just as important as what you eat. Muscles are most receptive to re-fuelling in the first half an hour or so immediately after exercise, so eat or drink something rich in carbohydrates as soon as possible after exercise. Fruit, freshly squeezed fruit juice diluted with water and sports drinks designed specifically for glycogen re-fuelling are ideal.

FLUID AND EXERCISE

Muscle is 75 percent water and a loss of just 3 per cent of this can cause the muscle to lose about 10 percent of its strength and 8 percent of its speed. Whenever the body is short of water, physical performance tends to decline. Lack of water also prevents the body producing enough sweat for adequate cooling, leading to a risk of overheating. This can also severely affect sports performance.

Everyone should drink at least 1.5 litres (3 pints) of plain water each day. Anyone who takes regular exercise will need to drink more than this to replace the fluid lost in sweat, as during prolonged exercise the body can lose up to 2 litres (4 pints) of fluid per hour.

Don't wait until you get thirsty before you drink. By the time you are thirsty, the chances are that you are already quite dehydrated. Get into the habit of drinking regularly throughout the day and at intervals during exercise itself if this is practical.

FOODS FOR BONE HEALTH

Healthy bones and joints are fundamental to a healthy, active life. Certain foods and nutrients contain the raw materials from which bones are composed and therefore can contribute to bone growth in childhood and continued bone and joint health in adult life. Other foods such as sugar can do the opposite, depleting the mineral content of bones and increasing the risk of bone weakness and thinning in later life.

GROWING BONES

Certain nutrients are necessary for healthy bone formation in children. Calcium is perhaps the most important bone-building nutrient, so children should get plenty of it in their diets – good sources are milk and cheese. Magnesium is another' important mineral for bone health. Many foods are rich in both calcium and magnesium. These include green leafy vegetables, sardines, mackerel, seafood and sesame seeds. Intake of sugar and fizzy drinks should be kept to a minimum as these can both cause loss of calcium from bones, leading to long-term bone weakness.

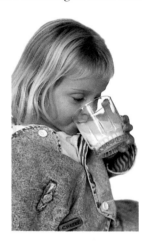

GOUT

Gout is a type of arthritis caused by an accumulation of uric acid in the body. Crystals of uric acid can form in a joint – usually the big toe – and lead to intense pain and inflammation. Uric acid is actually a breakdown product of a class of substances known as purines.
Fresh fruit and vegetables help to counter the effect of the uric acid in the body. Cherries are particularly helpful as they are rich in substances called proanthocyanidins, which help to neutralize uric acid and reduce inflammation of the joints.

FOODS TO AVOID FOR GOUT SUFFERERS

If you suffer from gout, you should avoid all foods that contain a high concentration of purines. These include meat, seafood, beans, peas, lentils, and organ meats such as liver and kidney.

OSTEOPOROSIS

Osteoporosis comes about when bone tissue is broken down faster than it is formed, so the bone becomes weakened, increasing the chances of fracture, especially in the spine and hips. Osteoporosis is much more common in women than men and is often related to the decline in the levels of oestrogen (one of the female sex hormones) after the menopause. Although osteoporosis is to some degree a natural part of the ageing process, there is a lot that can be done throughout life to help slow its progression.

PREVENTING OSTEOPOROSIS

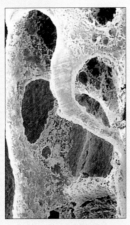

It is never too soon to start measures to prevent osteoporosis. The stronger your bones in youth, the more likely you are to retain bone strength in later life. Diet has an important part to play. Some foods can actually increase bone loss, while others supply the body with nutrients essential for healthy bone formation. Sugar, red meat and fizzy drinks all tend to speed up the rate at which calcium is lost from bone. Smoking also increases the risk of osteoporosis. Foods rich in the bone-building nutrients, calcium and magnesium, include green leafy vegetables, sardines, mackerel, seafood and sesame seeds. An important factor in bone strength is exercise. Studies have shown that gentle weight-bearing exercise reduces bone loss and may even increase bone density. Walking for 20-30 minutes each day will help to strengthen the bones. Other good forms of exercise include aerobics and light jogging.

THE EFFECTS OF OSTEOPOROSIS

In osteoporosis mineral loss from bone tissue leads to thinning and weakening of the bones. The photograph of bone tissue affected by osteoporosis (near right) clearly shows the dramatic reduction in bone density. This damaged bone is more fragile than the healthy bone shown (far right).

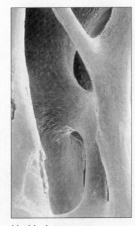

Osteoporosis damaged bone   Healthy bone

SLOWING AGEING

Many scientists around the world are engaged in studying the factors affecting ageing, with recent research focusing particularly on the role of damaging, destructive molecules called free radicals. These highly unstable molecules are generated in the body during the processes that create energy and there is evidence that they are at the heart of the ageing process.

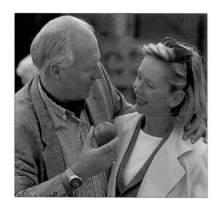

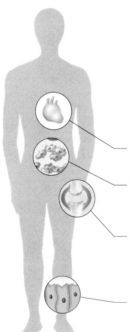

THE AGEING EFFECTS OF FREE RADICALS

Over the years, the presence of free radicals can cause widespread damage within the body, leading to increased susceptibility to various disorders and the outward signs of ageing. The effects of free radicals include:

■ **Damage to cell walls** which may predispose to heart disease and stroke.

■ **Damage to the internal mechanism of the cells** leading to genetic damage and a possible predisposition to cancer.

■ **Reduced immune function** leading to increased susceptibility to infection, increased risk of cancer and increased risk of inflammatory conditions such as rheumatoid arthritis.

■ **Damage to proteins in the skin** leading to a loss of tissue elasticity and function and an increase in skin wrinkling.

ANTI-OXIDANTS TO THE RESCUE

Fortunately, the body has ways of dealing with free radicals. Molecules called anti-oxidants can quench free radicals in the body (see page 88). So ageing is, to a degree, determined by the relative balance of free radicals to anti-oxidants – the greater the ratio of anti-oxidants to free radicals, the slower the ageing process. The main anti-oxidant nutrients are the vitamins A, C and E and the mineral selenium.

SOURCES OF ANTI-OXIDANTS

Anti-oxidant

Vitamin A and carotenoids such as beta-carotene are potent anti-oxidants with a particular role to play in protecting the lungs and skin.

Sources

Vitamin A – fish-liver oils, liver. Beta-carotene – green, orange and yellow fruit and vegetables such as carrots, cantaloupe melons, red, yellow and green peppers, apricots and mangoes.

Vitamin C is a powerful anti-oxidant and immune booster.

Oranges, grapefruit, lemons, blackcurrants, kiwi fruit and red, green and yellow peppers.

Vitamin E is an anti-oxidant and immune booster. It plays an important role in the prevention of heart disease.

Vegetable oils and some margarines, nuts (such as almonds or peanuts), seeds and wheatgerm.

Selenium is a powerful anti-oxidant which may help to reduce the risk of cancer.

Meat and organ meats, fish, shellfish, butter, citrus fruits, avocado pears and wholegrains.

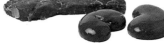

MENOPAUSE

During the reproductive years, a woman's cycle is regulated by a variety of hormones, the most important of which are oestrogen and progesterone. Around the time of menopause, the production of these hormones reduces dramatically, and this can give rise to a number of symptoms including night sweats, hot flushes, mood disturbance and loss of libido. The hormonal changes that accompany menopause are also associated with an increase in risk of certain medical conditions such as raised blood cholesterol, heart disease and osteoporosis.

REPLACING OESTROGEN THROUGH DIET

Certain dietary changes may help women during and after the time of menopause. Soya products such as tofu and soya milk may help to reduce hot flushes because they contain compounds that have oestrogen-like activity in the body. Countries in which large quantities of soya products are consumed in the diet (such as Japan) have low incidences of menopausal symptoms such as hot flushes among middle-aged women.

FOODS FOR ENERGY

There are four main categories of foods that are important for sustained energy release. This may be because of the quality of the energy-giving "fuel" they provide and/or because they contain nutrients that play vital roles in the processes that support energy production and activity in the body.

FRESH FRUIT

Fruit provides a ready supply of carbohydrate for conversion into energy in the body.

■ Rich in the mineral potassium, important for proper nerve and muscle function.

■ High in water, which has an essential role to play in almost all body processes.

■ Easily digested – so it does not sap the body of energy.

■ Generally releases sugar quite slowly into the bloodstream, helping to maintain blood sugar stability.

FRESH VEGETABLES

Some – mainly root vegetables such as potatoes, carrots and parsnips – provide a ready supply of carbohydrate for immediate conversion into energy in the body. Others – the green leafy vegetables – are rich in calcium and magnesium and play an important role in nerve and muscle function.

■ Rich in the mineral potassium, which has an important role in nerve and muscle function.

■ High in water, which is essential for almost all body processes.

■ Easily digested – so they do not sap the body of energy.

■ Generally release sugar quite slowly into the bloodstream, helping to maintain blood sugar stability.

■ Some (mainly the green leafy vegetables) are rich in iron and folic acid, both essential for healthy red blood cell formation.

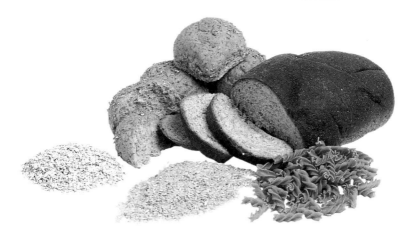

WHOLEGRAIN STARCHES

These provide a ready supply of carbohydrate for conversion into energy in the body.

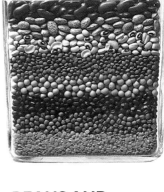

- Generally release sugar quite slowly into the bloodstream, helping to maintain blood sugar stability.
- Rich in B vitamins that play a role in the reactions that convert food into energy.
- Rich in chromium, essential for sugar metabolism and blood sugar stability.
- Rich in iron and folic acid, both essential for healthy red blood cell formation.

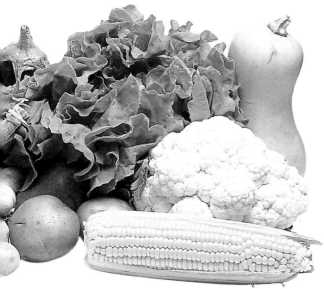

BEANS AND PULSES

These contain a high proportion of carbohydrate for conversion into energy in the body.

- Generally release sugar slowly into the bloodstream, helping to maintain blood sugar stability.
- Rich in B vitamins that are needed to convert food into energy in the body.

THE ENERGY SAPPERS

While some foods have a positive effect on general levels of energy and vitality in the body, there are undoubtedly some that have quite the opposite effect. Some foods are renowned for their energy-sapping ability, the main culprits being coffee, tea, chocolate, soft drinks, sugar and alcohol.

CAFFEINE

Caffeine in the diet comes from a variety of sources including coffee, tea and some soft drinks. Chocolate also contains caffeine-like substances that have a similar effect on the body. While caffeine can certainly improve energy levels in the short term, the boost is normally followed by a period of increased fatigue. Often, caffeinated soft drink, coffee and tea drinkers find that they become dependent on a certain level of consumption to maintain their energy levels. Excess caffeine consumption can lead to problems such as palpitations, anxiety and insomnia.

SUGARY FOOD AND DRINKS

The consumption of high-sugar foods and drinks, such as confectionery, biscuits, cakes and soft drinks, usually spells disaster for energy levels. These foods cause rapid rises in blood sugar which can cause the body to over-compensate, leading to problems with low blood sugar (hypoglycaemia) and low levels of physical and mental energy later on. In the long term, sugar may deplete the body of nutrients with an important part to play in the generation of energy in the body. Reduce your cravings for sugary snacks by ensuring you eat regular meals, thereby avoiding low blood sugar. If you need a snack, choose a low sugar alternative.

ALCOHOL

Alcohol can contribute to lethargy even when intoxication has worn off. Alcohol releases sugar rapidly into the bloodstream and may therefore also lead to problems with low blood sugar later. Many alcoholic beverages contain substances called congeners that contribute to hangovers and also deplete the body of energy. Try some of the alternative drinks suggested in the box. Or, if you don't want to cut out alcohol altogether, try diluting wine with water or adding extra non-alcoholic mixers to spirits.

ENERGY CONSERVING ALTERNATIVES

No caffeine, no alcohol drinks	Low-sugar snacks
■ Herb and fruit teas	■ Fresh fruit
■ Fruit juices	■ Wholemeal crackers
■ Spring water	■ Rice cakes
■ Sparkling herb drinks	■ Nuts and seeds
	■ Raw vegetables

EATING FOR A HEALTHY HEART

Heart disease is the leading cause of death in the developed world. Although heart disease is often thought of as a predominantly male condition, it is now the number one killer of women as well as men. According to the World Health Organization, 25 per cent of the 11 million deaths that occur in western society each year are due to heart disease. The good news is that a wealth of evidence exists to show that there is a lot we can do to prevent heart problems, and adjustments to eating habits are among the most beneficial measures.

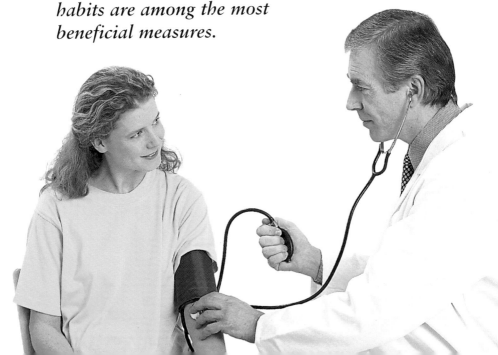

WHAT IS HEART DISEASE?

The heart is a muscular pump, about the size of a fist, situated in the centre of the chest between the lungs. Its function is to pump blood around the body so that essential substances such as oxygen and nutrients can be transported to every part. The blood is carried to the organs of the body in vessels called arteries, returning to the heart in vessels called veins.

2

Heart

Lungs

Veins (blue) carry deoxy-genated blood back to the heart and lungs.

Arteries (red) transport oxygenated blood away from the heart and lungs to every part of the body.

THE SUPPLY OF BLOOD TO THE HEART MUSCLE

Every organ and tissue in the body needs a blood supply, and the heart is no exception. The heart muscle is supplied with oxygenated blood by the three coronary arteries. If any of these vessels becomes clogged, a tiny blood clot (thrombus) is often all that it takes to cause a complete blockage of the artery. A heart attack is the result of such a blockage in a coronary artery, causing some of the heart muscle to die. The greater the area of damage, the higher the risk of death becomes.

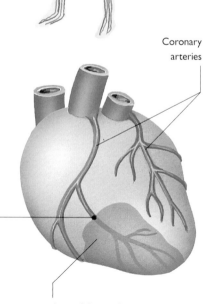

Coronary arteries

Blockage caused by a blood clot lodging in a coronary artery that has become narrowed as a result of fat deposits.

Area of damaged muscle that has been deprived of oxygenated blood during a heart attack.

FAT AND THE LINK WITH HEART DISEASE

Fat is transported around the body in the form of cholesterol and many experts regard high blood cholesterol as one of the most important risk factors for developing heart disease. Anyone can develop a high cholesterol level regardless of age, sex or race and, because there are no obvious warning signs, we cannot be sure whether or not we have a problem unless our cholesterol level is measured. However, diet can be effective in bringing cholesterol down, and this may reduce our risk of heart disease in the long term.

WHERE DOES CHOLESTEROL COME FROM?

Cholesterol in the body may be manufactured by the liver or it can come from the diet in the form of fat. Even relatively small changes in blood cholesterol may have a significant health benefit.

When fat is eaten, it is broken down in the gut and then passed into the bloodstream. Fat does not dissolve in blood and needs to be "packaged" before it can be transported around the body, so fat particles are wrapped in protein to make tiny parcels called lipoproteins (see page 31).

WHAT FUNCTION DO LIPOPROTEINS HAVE?

There are two basic types of lipoprotein: high density lipoprotein (HDL) and low density lipoprotein (LDL). LDL is transported around the body and is deposited at various sites including the coronary and cerebral arteries. LDL therefore plays a part in the development of atherosclerosis and so is sometimes referred to as "bad cholesterol". HDL, on the other hand, helps to remove fat from the body through the production of bile in the digestive tract. HDL seems to have the opposite effect to LDL and so is sometimes referred to as "good cholesterol".

HOW FAT IN THE BLOOD BLOCKS ARTERIES

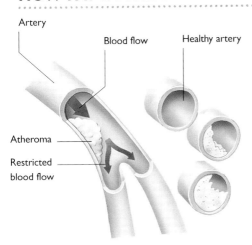

Artery

Blood flow   Healthy artery

Atheroma

Restricted
blood flow

When there are high levels of LDLs in the blood, fatty deposits tend to accumulate in the arteries. These fatty deposits or plaques are known as atheroma. Atheroma tends to form where the arteries branch, encouraged by turbulence in the blood flow. Severe atheroma in the coronary arteries, which supply the heart muscle, can restrict blood flow, causing chest pain known as angina pectoris. The presence of atheroma may also encourage the formation of blood clots (see left).

FAT AND HEART DISEASE

Fats in the diet can be divided broadly into three categories: saturated, mono-unsaturated and polyunsaturated. Diets high in saturated fats are strongly linked with heart disease. Saturated fats are found mainly in animal produce such as meat, eggs, whole milk, cheese, cream and butter. Foods such as chocolate, cakes and biscuits are also high in saturated fats.

2

THE MEDITERRANEAN DIET

Mono-unsaturated and polyunsaturated fats do not have the same strong links with heart disease as saturated fats, and many scientists believe they can actually help protect against this condition. Mono-unsaturated fats include olive oil, almond oil and avocado oil. A relatively high consumption of olive

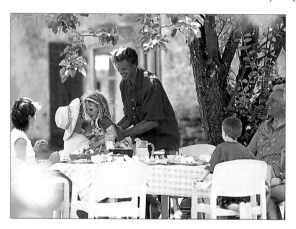

oil is thought to be one of the reasons why there is such a low incidence of heart disease in Mediterranean countries. Poly-unsaturated fats are found in fish, and are the main constituent of certain vegetable oils such as sunflower, safflower, sesame and grapeseed oils.

OAT BRAN TO REDUCE BLOOD CHOLESTEROL

Since the 1960s, some scientists have believed that oat bran may have cholesterol-lowering properties. Scientific studies have shown that oat bran can indeed be valuable in reducing blood cholesterol levels. The results showed that 5 grams of oat bran daily can lower blood cholesterol by up to 5 per cent and that this reduction is over and above that which could be achieved by a low cholesterol diet alone.

Oat bran can be eaten on its own or added to your usual breakfast cereal.

REDUCING CHOLESTEROL

In general we eat too much fat. You can reduce your cholesterol levels by limiting overall fat intake, while at the same time eating more unsaturated fats than the saturated variety. By following a few basic dietary guidelines, cholesterol levels can be lowered successfully.

■ Eat lean meat and cut off any visible fat. Red meats are generally higher in fat than poultry. One exception is venison, which is relatively lean compared to other red meats such as beef and lamb.

■ Eat poultry rather than red meats wherever possible. Poultry fat is mainly in the skin, so be sure to remove it.

■ Eat more fish. Oily fish such as herring, mackerel, tuna and trout are high in unsaturated fats that may protect against heart disease.

■ Moderate your consumption of eggs and dairy products such as cheese, whole milk, cream and butter. Choose low-fat varieties wherever possible, for example semi-skimmed or skimmed milk, low-fat cottage cheese and low-fat yoghurts. Whether margarines have any significant health benefit over butter is debatable and it is wisest to limit the use of both.

■ Moderate your consumption of chocolate, cakes and biscuits. Not only are these foods high in saturated fat, they also contain few nutrients or beneficial ingredients such as vitamins, minerals or fibre.

■ Avoid frying food as much as possible. Grilling, baking, steaming, boiling and poaching are all healthier ways to prepare food.

■ When you do use oil in cooking, make sure it is a vegetable oil. Cold-pressed oils which have had little or no refining are the healthiest of all oils.

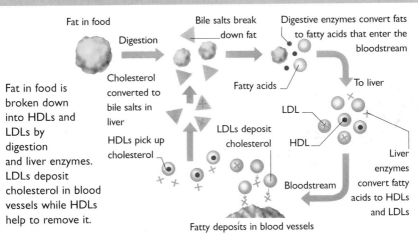

FROM DIETARY FAT TO BLOOD CHOLESTEROL

Fat in food

Digestion

Bile salts break down fat

Digestive enzymes convert fats to fatty acids that enter the bloodstream

Fat in food is broken down into HDLs and LDLs by digestion and liver enzymes. LDLs deposit cholesterol in blood vessels while HDLs help to remove it.

Cholesterol converted to bile salts in liver

HDLs pick up cholesterol

Fatty acids

LDLs deposit cholesterol

LDL

HDL

To liver

Liver enzymes convert fatty acids to HDLs and LDLs

Bloodstream

Fatty deposits in blood vessels

SUGAR AND THE HEART

When we eat sugar, some of it is converted in the body into a form of fat known as triglyceride, which does not have the same structure as cholesterol. Like cholesterol, however, it seems it does play a part in heart disease, although its exact significance is as yet uncertain.

THE IMPORTANCE OF TRIGLYCERIDES

2

Some research suggests that, in women, the triglyceride level is of greater significance than the cholesterol level. One study showed that women with the highest levels of triglyceride in their blood were seven times more likely to die from a heart attack compared to those with the lowest triglyceride levels. Some scientists and doctors believe that eating sugar has, through its effect on triglyceride levels, as important an effect on our risk of heart disease as fat.

SUGAR IN THE DIET

Because triglycerides come from sugar, it makes sense to cut down on the amount of sugar in the diet if you want to reduce the risk of heart disease. Some sources of sugar in the diet are obvious such as sweets, chocolate and other forms of confectionery, biscuits, cakes, soft drinks, sugared breakfast cereals and table sugar. These make up a sizeable proportion of sugar in the diet. However, sugar is also a common ingredient in many packaged and processed foods that are not sweet – so it is important to check the labels of the food you eat. The higher sugar is on the list of ingredients the more sugar that product contains. Canned vegetables, baked beans and "ready meals" often contain significant amounts of added sugar. Remember that sugar may not always be labelled as such. Some of the alternative terms used are listed in the box opposite.

Canned and processed
foods often contain
"hidden" sugar.

LESS FAT, MORE SUGAR

Many foods that claim to be "low in fat" or "virtually fat free" contain large amounts of sugar. Reducing the fat content of food can make it less palatable, so food manufacturers often get around this problem by adding extra sugar. Low-fat biscuits, cakes and ice-cream are all notable examples. The healthy solution is to change the types of food you eat, instead of trying to find healthy versions of basically unhealthy foods. For example, have a banana instead of a biscuit when you need a snack or choose unsweetened yoghurt instead of ice-cream.

ARTIFICIAL SWEETENERS

Artificial sweeteners such as saccharin and aspartame are now in widespread use as an alternative to sugar in many foodstuffs. Unlike sugar, artificial sweeteners contain few or no calories and do not raise triglyceride levels in the blood. However, artificial sweeteners may have other adverse effects in the body. Saccharin has been shown to cause tumours in laboratory animals and aspartame is known to change the levels of chemicals in the brain, which may lead to mood and sleep disturbances.

DOING WITHOUT SUGAR

There is some scientific evidence to suggest that consuming artificial sweeteners may actually encourage us to eat more food in the long term by enouraging the taste for sweetness and the expectation of an instant rise in blood sugar levels. So, while it is clearly a good idea to cut down on sugar, artificial sweeteners are probably not a healthy alternative. Should you need to add some sweetness to a dish, try some of the suggestions on page 107.

2

LABELLING SUGAR AND SUGAR SUBSTITUTES

Make sure you know the real content of the foods you buy by being aware of the different types of sugar and sweeteners used by food manufacturers. Look out for the following alternative names for sweetening agents when you check the ingredients listing of packaged foods.

Sugars

Dextrose
Fructose
Glucose
Lactose
Maltose
Sucrose

Sweeteners

Aspartame
Saccharin
Sorbitol

ASPARTAME AND PHENYLKETONURIA

The widely used artificial sweetener aspartame may pose special problems for individuals suffering from a rare medical condition known as phenylketonuria (PKU). People with this condition lack an enzyme which converts the amino acid phenylalanine into tyrosine (another amino acid). In children, the build-up of phenylalanine in the blood can cause problems with the development of the brain and nervous system. Because aspartame contains phenylalanine, it is especially important for PKU sufferers to avoid it.

SALT AND THE HEART

Salt is believed to increase the risk of heart disease by increasing blood pressure. Although for many years debate has raged in scientific circles about the relative importance of salt in high blood pressure, the latest evidence would suggest that it is, indeed, an important factor.

High blood pressure is an important risk factor for heart disease and affects about one in ten people. Contrary to popular opinion, high blood pressure (hypertension) rarely gives rise to symptoms and sufferers are therefore unaware that they may have a problem – so regular blood pressure checks are important.

NEW RESEARCH

One recent scientific study showed that salt has an important impact on the risk of high blood pressure and heart disease and that the effect of salt on our health is greater than had been previously supposed.

Scientific research has estimated that if everyone cut their salt intake by 30 per cent, there would be a 16 per cent fall in deaths due to heart disease and the number of people requiring treatment for high blood pressure would be halved. Cutting salt consumption by 60 percent would lead to a 30 per cent reduction in deaths due to heart disease and an 80 per cent reduction in the number of people requiring treatment for high blood pressure.

WHAT IS HIGH BLOOD PRESSURE?

Blood pressure measurement consists of two readings. The higher reading is known as the systolic pressure and measures pressure created by the contraction of the heart muscle. The lower reading, known as diastolic pressure, is taken when the heart muscle is relaxed. If either measurement is higher than normal, treatment for high blood pressure (hypertension) is usually advised. Blood pressure is usually best taken when you are rested and relaxed. This is because exercise and stress can raise blood pressure by up to 20mmHg on both readings giving an unrepresentative result.

Systolic	mmHg	Diastolic
	160	
	155	
	150	
	145	
High	140	
	135	
High normal	130	
Normal	125	
	120	
	115	
	110	
	105	
	100	
	95	
	90	High
	85	High normal
	80	Normal
	75	
	70	

REDUCING SALT IN THE DIET

Salt in the diet basically comes in two forms; salt we add during cooking or at the table, and salt already present in food, usually processed. To make valuable reductions in your intake, consider these suggestions:

■ To reduce salt consumption by 30 per cent, don't add salt during cooking or at the table.

■ To reduce salt consumption by 60 per cent, don't add salt during cooking or at the table or eat processed foods with salt added.

■ Try some of the alternative flavourings suggested on page 106.

2

IS SEA SALT BETTER THAN ORDINARY SALT?

Salt can be found in most supermarkets in a variety of forms including table salt, rock salt and sea salt. The sodium content of each of these forms of salt is virtually identical. Because it is the sodium which is the harmful element in salt, from a health point of view, any benefit one form of salt may have over any other is likely to be minimal.

FOODS WITH ADDED SALT

All of these food types are likely to have significant amounts of salt already added to them, and so are best avoided. Wherever possible, read the ingredients labels on foods to ascertain the salt content.

■ Bacon, ham, salt beef, sausages, burgers, pies and canned meat.

■ Fish fingers, shellfish, smoked and canned fish.

■ Instant meals.

■ Some breakfast cereals including high fibre cereals described as "healthy".

■ Canned and packet soups and sauces.

■ Stock cubes and yeast extracts.

■ Butter (except unsalted), margarine and cheese.

■ Crisps, salted nuts and similar snacks.

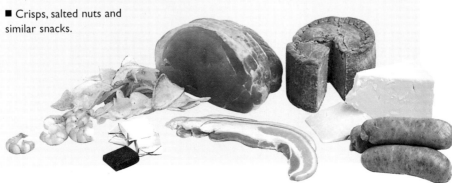

PREVENTING DAMAGE

Oxygen is essential for life and is involved in countless reactions within our body every day. However, these life-sustaining processes also produce dangerous by-products. During such chemical reactions, free radicals molecules can be formed, accelerating the processes that lead to heart disease. The cells that line the coronary arteries try to heal themselves by plugging up the damage caused by free radicals with cholesterol and blood clots, thus increasing the risk of heart attack.

2

FREE RADICALS AND THE ROLE OF ANTI-OXIDANTS

Free radicals are molecules released as a natural by-product of normal cell activity. It is now thought that these molecules can cause considerable damage to the body if they accumulate excessively. In particular, they are believed to attack the nucleus of body cells. Damage to the cells lining the blood vessels can lead to an increase tendency for fatty deposits. Free radicals also seem to play a role in the development of cancer (page 88). However, research has also shown that anti-oxidants in the diet can neutralize the damaging activity of free radicals.

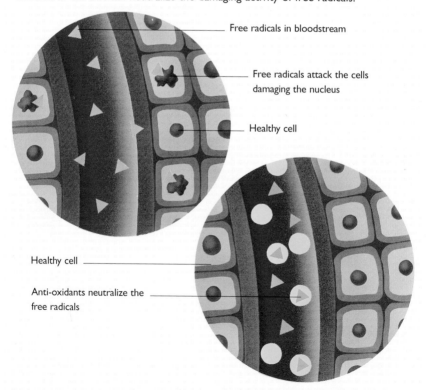

Free radicals in bloodstream

Free radicals attack the cells damaging the nucleus

Healthy cell

Healthy cell

Anti-oxidants neutralize the free radicals

ANTI-OXIDANTS AND THE HEART

The damaging effects of free radicals on the heart and blood vessels are neutralized by the action of the anti-oxidant nutrients such as beta-carotene, vitamins A, C and E and selenium, a mineral: and there is now much evidence to suggest that a diet rich in anti-oxidants may help protect against heart disease. Foods that contain high levels of these nutrients include fresh fruit, vegetables and wholegrains such as wholegrain bread, brown rice and wholewheat pasta. Eating an abundance of these foods in the diet can reduce your risk of developing heart disease.

In addition to eating a diet rich in anti-oxidant nutrients, it may also be of benefit to take them as a dietary supplement. Suitable supplements can be found in good health food stores and pharmacies. It is important to remember, however, that vitamin and mineral pills are supplements to and not substitutes for a healthy diet.

2

HEALTHY FATS

Certain healthy fats in the diet can also help reduce the risk of heart disease. Essential fats contained in oily fish, olive oil and pumpkin, sunflower and sesame seeds can help protect against atherosclerosis and may also help to thin the blood. Concentrated fish oil supplements are rich in omega-3 fatty acids and may confer additional benefit in the long term. The normal dose is 1 gram taken two or three times a day.

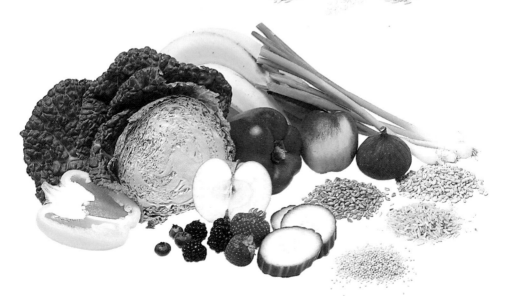

Fresh fruit and vegetables and wholegrains are essential sources of anti-oxidants.

COOKING FOR THE HEART

The effect of food on the health of our heart is not only determined by the nutritional content of the food, but the way in which it is prepared. The cooking methods and recipes you choose have a particular impact on the amount of fat in the diet. It may take a little time to adjust to a "heart healthy" way of cooking, but with imagination and careful selection of ingredients, you can provide yourself and your family with a range of tasty alternatives.

2

DONT'S

- Don't use full-fat milk or cream in cooking.

- Don't add butter to boiled or steamed vegetables.

- Don't make red meat the chief component of your meals.

- Don't use recipes that contain large amounts of cheese.

- Don't make pre-prepared dishes a regular part of your meals. They often contain "hidden" salt and sugar.

- Don't serve pastries and biscuits, which often contain a high proportion of fat.

- Don't choose fatty meat or high fat meat products such as sausages and salami.

- Don't buy pre-basted meat which is often injected with fat.

- Don't fry foods.

- Don't add large amounts of fat or oil in cooking.

- Don't use salad dressings or mayonnaises that are usually high in fat.

Deep-fat frying adds large quantities of damaging fats to foods.

Fried fish is high in fats. The breadcrumb coating holds added fat, increasing the health risk.

Chips absorb a large amount of fat in cooking. The fact that the fat is also heated to high temperatures may also increase the health risk.

Bread with butter adds to the fat overload.

DO'S

- Replace full-fat milk with skimmed milk in all recipes.

- Replace cream with low-fat crème fraîche or low-fat yoghurt.

- Mix mayonnaise half and half with low-fat yoghurt. This mixture can be used as a dressing for potato salad and other salad dishes. Mustard is a good alternative to mayonnaise in sandwiches.

- Choose low-fat cheeses in preference to full-fat soft or hard cheeses.

- Reduce the amount of salt you add to all recipes.

- Sauté vegetables in stock or wine instead of butter or oil.

- Serve smaller portions of high-fat foods such as meat and dairy produce while increasing the portion size of low-fat foods such as steamed vegetables, potatoes, pasta and rice.

- Replace pastries and cream-laden desserts with fresh fruit.

- Reduce the amount of fat and oil you use in cooking.

- Choose lean cuts of meat and trim off the fat before cooking.

- Remove the skin from poultry before cooking.

- Roast, grill, bake or stew meat and fish.

- Chill meat stews and soups so that the fat rises to the top and solidifies. This can then be spooned off and discarded.

- Use non-stick cookware to reduce the need for oil and fat during cooking.

- Use fat-free or low-fat salad dressings such as vinegar, lemon juice or low-fat yoghurt.

2

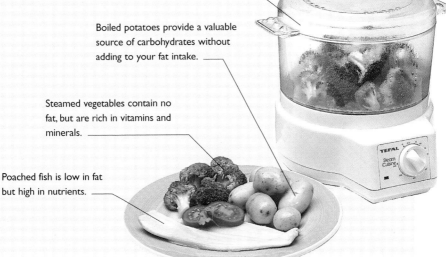

Steaming is one of the best ways of cooking vegetables as it preserves a high proportion of vitamins.

Boiled potatoes provide a valuable source of carbohydrates without adding to your fat intake.

Steamed vegetables contain no fat, but are rich in vitamins and minerals.

Poached fish is low in fat but high in nutrients.

ALCOHOL AND THE HEART

Most of us are familiar with the idea that a moderate amount of alcohol may be good for us. More and more research is being done that tends to support this idea. Many studies have shown that male and female abstainers have a higher risk of developing heart disease than people who consume moderate amounts. The precise explanation for this remains unclear, although it is now known that alcohol raises the levels of high-density lipoproteins (see page 29), which are beneficial to health, by about 15 per cent on average, and reduces the tendency of the blood to clot. Too much alcohol, however, can actually increase the clotting tendency of blood.

THE BENEFITS OF ALCOHOL

Moderate alcohol consumption is also associated with reduced death rate from all causes. If a graph is plotted of death against alcohol consumption, the result is a J-shaped curve. On the left are the teetotallers who are at increased risk, while on the right, those who consume excessive amounts of alcohol are at high risk, too. However, the curve has a wide base, and it takes quite a lot of alcohol before a drinker's risk of mortality equals that of the teetotaller.

ADVANTAGES OF MODERATE ALCOHOL CONSUMPTION

Risk of death

Moderate risk   Low risk   Moderate risk   High risk

Units of alcohol per week

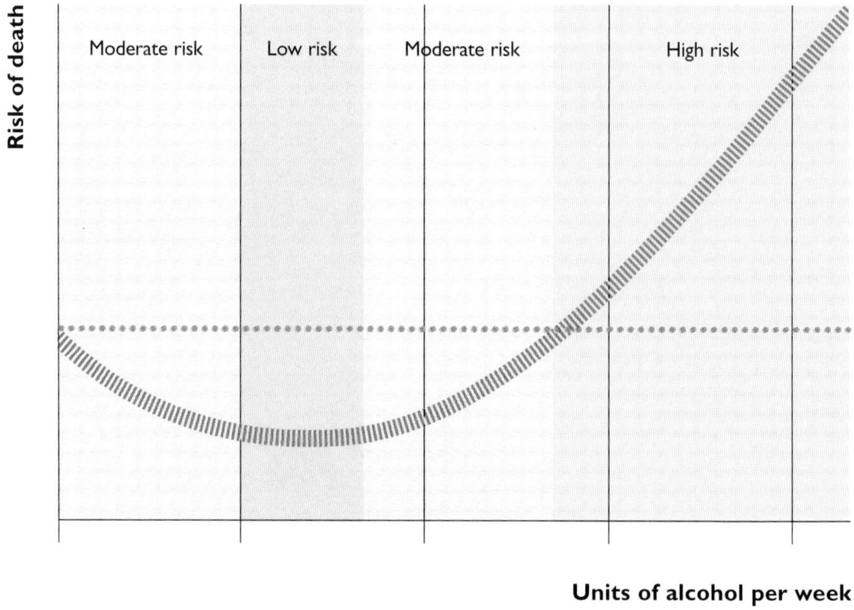

WHAT IS A SAFE LEVEL?

Moderate alcohol consumption is associated with a reduced risk of stroke, and elderly moderate drinkers retain better brain function and have denser bones than abstainers or heavy drinkers. Although the benefits of alcohol in moderation are widely accepted, scientists have not been able to agree on what actually constitutes the safest level. A recent Danish study put the level at one to six units per week, while an American study has calculated the safe level to be about 10 units per week. In the United Kingdom, government guidelines suggest an upper limit of 28 units for men and 21 units for women, although many doctors feel that these levels are too high.

DETERMINING THE RIGHT LEVEL FOR YOU

In the light of such evidence, what conclusions can be drawn? One fact which appears not to be in dispute is that moderate alcohol consumption can help protect against heart disease and reduce overall mortality rates. However, the optimum level of drinking probably varies from individual to individual. Overall, the message seems to be: drink sensibly with food, spread your drinking over the whole week, and avoid getting drunk.

Warning!

No possible long-term health benefits from moderate alcohol consumption are worth the immediate risks associated with irresponsible drinking.

■ Remember – never drink if you intend to drive or operate dangerous machinery.

■ Excessive alcohol consumption has serious health consequences, from high blood pressure to cirrhosis of the liver and cancer as well as economic and social repercussions.

■ If you are taking medication, ask your doctor before drinking alcohol.

2

MEASURING ALCOHOL INTAKE

Alcohol consumption is usually measured in units of alcohol per week, where a unit of alcohol is equivalent to one glass of wine, a single measure of spirits, or half a pint (about 25cl) of beer.

Each of these drinks contains one unit of alcohol.

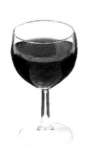

1 small glass of wine

1 small measure of spirits

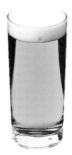

1 small glass of beer

MEALS FOR THE HEART

A good diet that will ensure a healthy heart can also be quite delicious. The emphasis should be on fresh fruit and vegetables, pulses, wholegrains, and a low intake of fat, sugar and salt. The meal suggestions outlined here are simply a guide. By choosing equivalent foods to suit your taste, it is possible to eat a healthy diet that is both varied and interesting.

BREAKFASTS FOR A HEALTHY HEART

Breakfasts should provide an energy boost and vitamins and other nutrients to help you start the day full of vitality. However, for most people leading hurried lifestyles it also needs to be a meal with a minimum of preparation. For those with a particular concern for the health of the heart, a low-fat breakfast based around fruit and wholegrain cereals is ideal.

■ Low-sugar or no-sugar breakfast cereal based on oats, wheat, corn or rice, skimmed milk, fruit and seeds (sesame, sunflower or pumpkin).

■ Wholegrain rye or wheat-based bread or toast with "no added sugar" jam.

■ Fresh fruit salad with low-fat natural yoghurt.

■ Blended fruit smoothie made with strawberries, low-fat yoghurt, ice and a small amount of honey.

■ Dried fruit compote with fresh orange segments with low-fat natural yoghurt or fromage frais.

■ Oat-bran muffin with a piece of fresh fruit.

■ No-added sugar muesli with low-fat natural yoghurt.

■ Porridge made with skimmed milk topped with dried or fresh fruit.

■ Wholegrain toast with cottage cheese, fresh fruit.

■ Drop pancakes with unsweetened apple purée and honey.

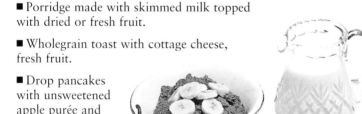

LUNCHES FOR A HEALTHY HEART

For busy working people lunch is seldom a leisurely, large meal. But it is important to ensure that your energy and vitamin stores are topped up. Avoid the temptation to opt for fat- and salt-laden "fast foods" such as chips and burgers. There are plenty of nutritious low-fat alternatives to try. Follow your main course with one of the dessert suggestions below.

- Fresh vegetable soup and rye crackers.

- Skinless chicken salad sandwich on wholegrain rye or wheat bread.

- Skinless chicken or tuna salad dressed with extra virgin olive oil and lemon juice.

- Jacket potato filled with plain or flavoured cottage cheese, tuna and sweetcorn or reduced fat crème fraîche, and a side salad.

- Sardines on wholegrain rye or wheat toast with grilled tomatoes.

- Grilled fish cakes (made with white fish, salmon or tuna) with mixed salad or steamed vegetables.

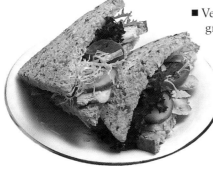

- Vegeburger, chicken or tuna with char-grilled vegetables, served in pitta bread.

- Grilled mackerel or herring coated in oatmeal with steamed vegetables.

- Lentil or bean salad with wholegrain bread and green leaf salad.

DESSERT SUGGESTIONS

- Fresh fruit.
- Low-fat yoghurt.
- Unsweetened fruit crumble, with oat or muesli topping.
- Fresh or canned fruit purée mixed with low-fat natural yoghurt or fromage frais.
- Fresh fruit topped with natural low-fat yoghurt and sprinkled with brown sugar and grilled until caramelized.
- Baked apples with low-fat natural yoghurt.

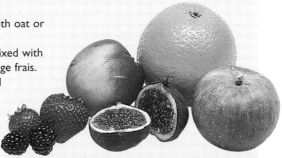

continued ▶

SUPPERS FOR A HEALTHY HEART

The evening is often a time when it is convenient to cook a more elaborate meal than you can in the day. Concentrate on choosing fresh ingredients. Your heart will benefit from plenty of vegetables, cooked lightly to preserve their vitamin content, and plainly cooked fish, made flavoursome with herbs and spices, instead of salt. Alternatively, try dishes based around wholegrain pasta or pulses, accompanied by a salad. Follow with one of the dessert suggestions on the previous page.

- Grilled or poached trout or salmon with steamed vegetables and boiled new potatoes in their skins.

- Fish casserole with baked potato and steamed vegetables.

- Pasta with tomato-based sauce with salad dressed with extra virgin olive oil and sesame seeds.

- Chicken casserole with brown rice and steamed green vegetables.

- Grilled prawn kebabs with a side salad.

- Chicken satay and raw vegetable sticks with yoghurt-based or thin peanut sauce.

- Grilled vegetables brushed with extra virgin olive oil, served with brown rice and a side salad.

- Wholewheat pasta with a sauce made from reduced-fat crème fraîche and seafood or mushrooms.

- Baked cod or other white fish with wholegrain breadcrumb and herb topping and grilled tomatoes and steamed vegetables.

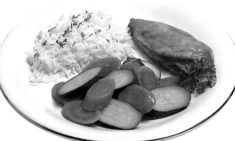

- Lentil or bean casserole and steamed vegetables.

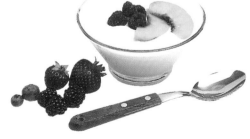

EATING FOR DIGESTIVE HEALTH

The digestive tract is responsible for the digestion and absorption of food and the elimination of waste material at the other end. Gut-related disorders are common and up to 80 percent of individuals suffer from

3

symptoms that are a sign of digestive ill-health. Dietary adjustments can provide a simple and effective remedy for a wide range of digestive symptoms, including indigestion, constipation and irritable bowel syndrome. Improving the health of the digestive system by changing your eating habits will also lead to an overall improvement in your health as nutrients are more effectively absorbed.

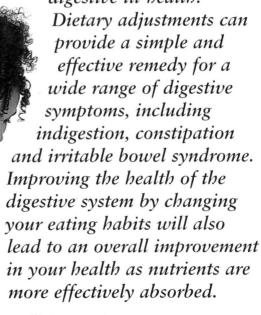

DIGESTION AT WORK

The digestive tract is a tube several metres long that begins at the mouth and runs to the anus at the other end. It has eight main components: the mouth, the oesophagus, the stomach, the small and large intestines, the pancreas, the gallbladder and the liver. Each part of the digestive tract has a role to play in breaking down the food we eat so that it can be absorbed and used by the body.

3

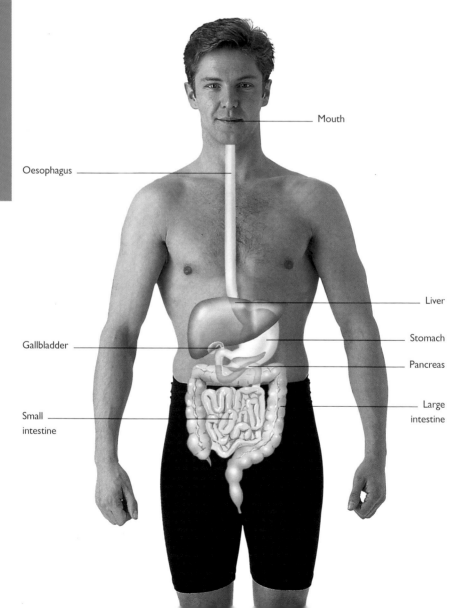

Mouth

Oesophagus

Liver

Gallbladder

Stomach

Pancreas

Small intestine

Large intestine

THE MOUTH

Digestion of food starts in the mouth and the very act of chewing stimulates the secretion of digestive juices lower down in the gut. Chewing also mixes food with saliva which contains an enzyme called amylase that starts the digestion of starchy foods such as bread, potatoes, rice and pasta. Breaking up the food increases the efficiency of digestion by giving digestive enzymes the opportunity to penetrate the food more effectively.

THE STOMACH

After the food has been swallowed, it travels down a tube called the oesophagus which transports it to the stomach. The stomach secretes acid, which starts the process of digestion of protein-based foods such as meat, fish and dairy products. The lining of the stomach is protected from the action of the acid by a thick coat of mucus.

THE SMALL INTESTINE AND PANCREAS

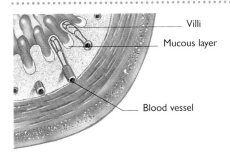

Villi

Mucous layer

Blood vessel

3

After it leaves the stomach, food passes into the small intestine, where the action of more enzymes continues the digestive process. Some of these are produced in the wall of the gut itself, while others are secreted by the pancreas. Bile, a digestive juice that assists the digestion of fats, also enters the small intestine (see The liver and gallbladder below). Nutrients are absorbed through the lining of the small intestine.

THE LARGE INTESTINE

After food has been absorbed from the small intestine into the bloodstream, the remainder passes into the large intestine. This waste matter is very liquid but becomes gradually more solid as water is absorbed through the wall of the large intestine back into the body. The end product is faeces, eliminated from the body via the rectum and anus.

THE LIVER AND GALLBLADDER

The food molecules that are absorbed through the gut all pass into the bloodstream and are carried to the liver. Here, some food molecules are broken down still further while others are converted into forms that can be stored as fuel around the body. The gallbladder is a small sac-like structure which sits underneath the liver. Its function is to store bile, produced in the liver, which it then secretes into the small intestine.

POOR DIGESTION

Ideally, the digestive process should occur swiftly and efficiently so that optimum nutritional value is obtained from the food we eat. If digestion is too slow, undigested food may ferment in the digestive tract, leading to discomfort and poor absorption of nutrients.

CAUSES OF POOR DIGESTION

■ **Failure to chew thoroughly,** usually due to eating too quickly. Chewing has a very important part to play in the digestive process. Failure to chew thoroughly can impair digestion and reduce the efficiency of the other elements of the digestive process.

■ **Eating large meals.** The digestive system can only do so much at one time. The bigger the meal you eat, the less able the digestive system will be to digest it completely.

■ **Drinking large volumes of liquid with meals.** Drinking too much fluid with meals dilutes the secretions (acid, digestive enzymes and bile) that are responsible for the digestive process. The dilution of these secretions impairs their efficiency and disrupts the digestive process.

■ **Late meals.** The digestive processes wind down at the end of the day so eating late at night is a common cause of digestive problems.

■ **Stress.** It is well known that stress impairs the digestive process.

■ **Low stomach acid/digestive enzyme secretion.** Some individuals do not produce sufficient amounts of stomach acid and/or digestive enzymes for efficient digestion.

SYMPTOMS OF POOR DIGESTION

■ **Lack of energy.** Inefficiently digested food is unlikely to be absorbed into the bloodstream. Much of it is therefore trapped in the gut, instead of being transported to the body's cells for the generation of energy.

■ **Nutritional deficiencies.** The vitamins and minerals essential for life come via our diet, so poor digestion and absorption of food are very likely to lead to multiple nutritional deficiencies. Such deficiencies may have far-reaching, long-term consequences, from fatigue to increased risk of conditions such as heart disease and cancer.

■ **Digestive discomfort.** If the digestive system is inefficient, undigested or partially digested food can be left to ferment in the gut. This can lead to problems with wind production – burping and flatulence – as well as bloating and abdominal discomfort.

■ **Altered bowel habit.** Poor digestion quite commonly leads to problems with constipation, loose bowels and occasionally a combination of both.

WHAT IS INDIGESTION?

Indigestion is the term commonly used to describe abdominal discomfort that occurs after eating. The pain is typically felt in the middle of the upper abdomen. Other common symptoms include nausea, bloating and excessive burping. Common causes of indigestion include gastritis (an inflammation in the lining of the stomach), or an ulcer in the stomach or the first part of the small intestine called the duodenum (see page 51). The contributing factors include excess or low stomach acidity, inadequate chewing of food and the consumption of large meals.

DO'S AND DON'TS FOR PREVENTING INDIGESTION

DO

■ **Chew food thoroughly** Each mouthful of food should be chewed 20-30 times.

■ **Eat little and often** Because large meals may overload the digestive system, it makes sense to avoid eating too much at one time.

■ **Make your meals appetizing** The anticipation of a tasty meal increases the secretion of digestive juices thereby promoting better digestion.

DON'T

■ **Don't eat late in the evening** Try not to eat later than about 8.00 pm.

■ **Don't drink with meals** Quench your thirst by drinking between meals instead and take no more than one small glass of fluid at mealtimes.

■ **Don't take over-the-counter indigestion remedies** except on the advice of your doctor. Antacids can actually reduce the efficiency of digestion.

■ **Don't eat while you are working** Keep mealtimes stress-free and avoid distractions such as reading or television while you are eating.

■ **Don't rush meals** Set aside sufficient time for your meals so that you can enjoy your food without hurry and relax for some minutes afterwards.

3

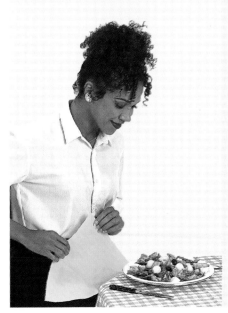

HEARTBURN AND ULCERS

There are several possible underlying causes of the discomfort after eating commonly known as indigestion. Heartburn is a particular type of burning pain in the centre of the upper abdomen, which may be caused by poor eating habits or by a weakness in the muscle that separates the abdomen from the chest. Peptic ulcers can also cause digestive discomfort. Changes in eating habits can help in both cases.

HEARTBURN

This condition is characterized by a sensation of burning and discomfort in the centre of the chest behind the breastbone (sternum). It is often worse when you bend or lie down. It is caused by the escape of acid from the stomach into the oesophagus. This may sometimes be the result of a hiatus hernia (below). Contributory factors may be excess or low stomach acidity, inadequate chewing of food and the consumption of large meals. Heartburn is also more likely at night, because lying down makes it easier for the stomach contents to escape into the oesophagus.

HIATUS HERNIA

When we swallow, food is carried down the oesophagus into the stomach but, just before it opens into the stomach, the oesophagus passes through a sheet of muscle called the diaphragm. In a hiatus hernia, part of the stomach is pushed up through the diaphragm, allowing acid in the stomach to escape into the oesophagus. This condition is known as "acid reflux", and typical symptoms include heartburn and digestive discomfort.

COMBATING ACID REFLUX

Dietary changes can be very effective in reducing the symptoms of acid reflux that occur with heartburn and hiatus hernia.

■ Avoid large meals, as the more food and drink you have in your stomach, the greater the risk of acid reflux. This is especially true at night, because lying down makes it much more likely that acid will escape from the stomach.

■ Eat your evening meal at least three hours before going to bed to allow most of the food you have eaten to pass out of the stomach before you retire.

■ Prop yourself up in bed with pillows. This may help to relieve nighttime discomfort.

■ Chew your food very thoroughly, and avoid drinking large quantities of fluid with meals.

■ Food combining is usually very effective in combating symptoms (see pages 52–53).

WHAT IS A PEPTIC ULCER

The lining of the gut is shielded from potentially damaging digestive secretions by a coating of protective mucus. Sometimes, this protective mechanism breaks down leading to the development of a raw area or ulcer. The majority of ulcers develop in the part of the gut just below the stomach called the duodenum, although they may also occur in the lining of the stomach. Peptic ulcers seem to be in part caused by the *Helicobacter pylori* bacterium. Symptoms may be similar to those of indigestion (page 49).

HEALING ULCERS THROUGH DIET

Dietary changes and certain nutritional supplements may promote ulcer healing and help prevent a recurrence of the problem. Avoid sugar, alcohol, coffee and tea as these all seem to increase the risk of developing an ulcer or to slow down its healing. A high-fibre diet seems to prevent recurrence of ulcers once they have healed so make sure your diet is rich in high-fibre foods such as oats, brown rice, fruit and vegetables.

MILK AND ULCERS

In the past it was thought that drinking a glass of milk was a good way to relieve the discomfort of a peptic ulcer. However, there is now evidence to suggest that milk actually encourages *Helicobacter pylori*, the bacterium that is now believed to be a major cause of ulcers. Ulcer sufferers should therefore avoid milky drinks.

3

PEPTIC ULCERS AND STRESS

Peptic ulcers may be related to a stressful lifestyle or may develop at a time in your life when you have been subjected to prolonged stress. Try to reduce any generalized sources of stress. Avoid hurried mealtimes, which discourage proper chewing and digestion and try to avoid working while you are eating.

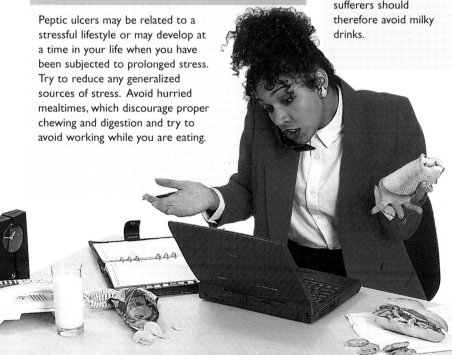

FOOD COMBINING

Foods are made up of several chemical constituents including proteins, starches, fats, vitamins, minerals, fibre and water. The common proteins in the diet can be found in animal products such as meat, fish, dairy products and eggs. The common starches in the diet are bread, rice, pasta, cereals and potatoes. Proteins and starches are very different chemically and are digested by different enzymes in the gut. Proteins are also initially digested in acid, while starches are digested in alkali – so quite the opposite. Some people have digestive systems that are unable to cope with protein/starch combinations, and this can lead to digestive problems that may be helped by food combining.

3

ORIGINS OF FOOD COMBINING

The concept of food combining as a way to better digestive and overall health was popularized in the 1930s by an American physician Dr William Howard Hay. Having improved his own health by practising the principles of food combining, he abandoned his career as a surgeon to promote his ideas and treat patients according to his dietary guidelines. The common name for food combining, the Hay Diet, is a tribute to the key work of Dr Hay in its development.

FOOD COMBINING IN PRACTICE

The basic principle of food combining is to avoid mixing protein and starch at the same meal. So each meal should consist of protein with "neutral" foods or starch with neutral foods. Neutral foods in food combining terms include most vegetables (potatoes are the chief exception) and pure fats and oils. It is thought that by separating protein and starch at each meal, the digestion of each type of food is enhanced.

MEAL SUGGESTIONS

With practice and experience you will develop a range of interesting food combining meal ideas of your own. But the following suggestions may be useful if you are new to food combining:

■ Meat or fish with salad or vegetables other than the potato.

■ Pasta with meatless tomato-based sauce and salad.

■ Vegetable curry and rice.

■ Baked potato, ratatouille and salad.

■ Meat stew with vegetables.

■ Avocado salad

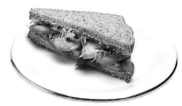

FOOD COMBINING GROUPS

Protein	Neutral	Starch
Any protein can be eaten with any neutral food		

Protein	Neutral	Starch
Meats	**All green and**	**Basic**
Beef	**root vegetables**	**carbohydrates**
Lamb	**except potatoes**	Bread
Chicken	Asparagus	Rice
Turkey	Aubergines	Pasta
Veal	Broccoli	Cereal
Venison	Brussels sprouts	Potatoes
Pork	Cabbage	
Bacon	Carrots	**Flour-based foods**
	Cauliflower	Pastries and pies
Fish	Celery	Cakes
Mackerel	Courgettes	Biscuits
Herring	Green beans	
Trout	Leeks	**Dried fruit**
Salmon	Mushrooms	Dates
Tuna	Onions	Figs
Cod	Parsnips	Currants
Plaice	Peas	Sultanas
Skate	Spinach	Raisins
	Turnips	
Shellfish		**Other fruit**
Prawns	**Salad vegetables**	Bananas
Cockles	Avocado	Mangoes
Mussels	Cucumber	
Oysters	Tomatoes	**Sweeteners**
Crab	Lettuce	Sugar
Lobster	Spring onions	Maple syrup
	Red and green peppers	Honey
Dairy products	Radishes	
Cheese		
Eggs	Nuts and seeds	
Milk		
Yoghurt	**Fats and oils**	
	Cream	
Vegetable proteins	Butter	
Soya beans	Extra virgin olive oil	
Soya bean curd (tofu)	Other vegetable oils	

Any starch can be eaten with any neutral food

FRESH FRUIT

In food combining terms, fresh fruit, other than bananas and mangos (see table above), is in a category of its own: it is neither protein nor starch, nor is it neutral. You should not eat fruit at mealtimes. It should be eaten on its own between meals.

COMBATING CONSTIPATION

Bowel regularity is very important for health and constipation can increase the risk of certain bowel conditions. In the long term, small pouches can develop in the wall of the lower part of the colon, known as diverticuli. These can sometimes become inflamed or infected with waste material and this, in turn, can give rise to pain on the left side of the abdomen. More serious complications such as bleeding and bowel perforation may also develop. Doctors refer to this condition as diverticular disease and its development is almost always related to long-standing constipation. Long-standing constipation can also increase the risk of cancer of the colon.

In the shorter term, if waste products are not eliminated efficiently from the body, harmful waste products can build up leading to problems such as fatigue, bad breath and poor skin health.

INCREASE YOUR FIBRE INTAKE

One essential ingredient for healthy bowel function is fibre. This indigestible material adds bulk to the food residues, thereby promoting the passage of waste materials through the intestines. High-fibre breakfast cereals based on wheat bran are often advised for people suffering from constipation. However, the fibre in these cereals is quite hard and scratchy and may actually irritate the delicate lining of the gut. The fibre found in oats, fresh fruit, vegetables and pulses is generally much kinder to the gut. For optimum bowel function, as well as to ensure adequate intake of vitamins and minerals, you should eat at least five servings of fruit or vegetables a day.

Warning!

A sudden change in bowel habit can sometimes be related to a potentially serious underlying condition. If you experience constipation after years of regularity, consult your doctor so that any underlying disease can be excluded.

LAXATIVES

Many individuals use laxatives based on substances such as sennakot to ensure regular bowel movements. Although these may temporarily relieve a constipation problem, many people become reliant on laxatives for their bowel function. Part of this is because laxatives may stimulate the gut abnormally – causing the gut to lose its ability to function normally. Laxatives also often contain agents that irritate the lining of the gut, which is not good for general digestive health. Ideally, any problem with constipation should be relieved as naturally as possible and the use of laxatives, especially in the long term, should be avoided.

USE NATURAL BULKING AGENTS

An effective and convenient way to increase fibre intake is to add a natural bulking agent to your diet. Take 1–2 dessertspoons of either psyllium husks or linseeds with water each day, or sprinkled over cereals, soups or salads.

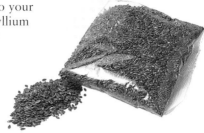

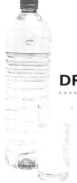

Linseeds are one of the most effective natural bulking agents.

DRINK MORE WATER

Apart from fibre, the other essential ingredient for bowel regularity is fluid. The best form of fluid for bowel health is water. Drink 1$\frac{1}{2}$–2 litres (3–4 pints) of still water each day. Alcohol can dehydrate the body and so actually make constipation worse.

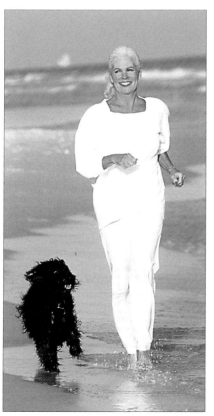

TAKE EXERCISE

3

Exercise can help relieve constipation, probably through the mechanical action of the abdominal muscles and diaphragm on the bowel. Aim to take 30 minutes' worth of aerobic exercise, such as brisk walking, light jogging, cycling, rowing, aerobics or aqua-aerobics, at least three or four times a week. Not only will regular exercise help to improve your bowel habit, but it will also benefit your overall health.

ALWAYS RESPOND TO THE CALL OF NATURE

Always respond promptly to the urge to open your bowels. Failure to do this on a regular basis may cause a suppression of the nerve impulses that are essential for defecation to take place. The long-term result may be persistent constipation.

IRRITABLE BOWEL

One condition that is being diagnosed more and more frequently is irritable bowel syndrome or IBS. IBS affects 10-20 per cent of the population in the western world and affects twice as many women as it does men. Although about 60 per cent of individuals attending a gastroenterology clinic suffer from IBS, conventional medicine has yet to find a definite cause or cure for this condition.

There are many possible contributory causes of irritable bowel syndrome and most are relatively harmless. However, some symptoms associated with the condition may be a sign of underlying disease and should be investigated by a doctor.

TYPICAL SYMPTOMS

Sufferers from irritable bowel syndrome may experience some or all of the following symptoms:

- Constipation or diarrhoea, or alternating constipation and diarrhoea.
- Bloating of the abdomen.
- Lower abdominal pain.
- Flatulence.

3

MUSCLE SPASM IN IRRITABLE BOWEL SYNDROME

Some sufferers from IBS experience disruption to the normally smooth contractions of the bowel. Irregular spasm of the muscles of the bowel wall causes cramping pains and interferes with the passage of food residues through the bowel, leading to constipation and/or diarrhoea.

Normal bowel
contractions

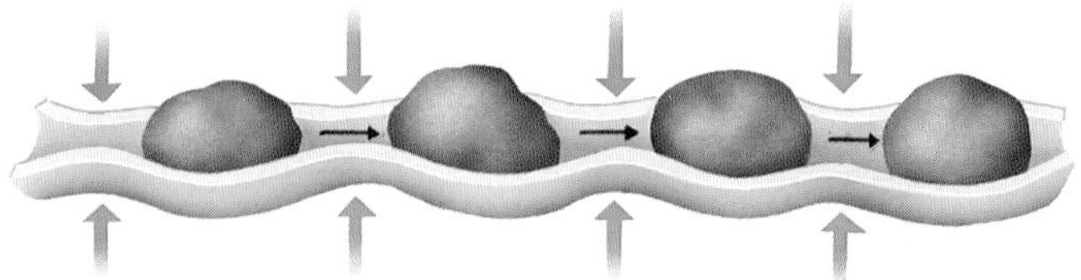

Irregular bowel
contractions

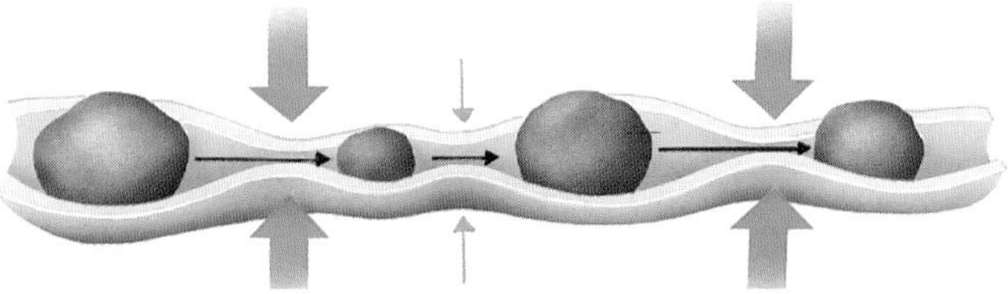

BACTERIAL ACTIVITY IN THE GUT

A major cause of IBS is an imbalance in the organisms that inhabit the gut. Quite often problems are related to an overgrowth of the yeast organism, candida. This organism tends to ferment food which leads to the bloating and wind characteristic of IBS. The secret to getting on top of yeast is to starve it out of the system. This means eliminating temporarily from the diet all foods that feed yeast or are inherently yeasty, mouldy or fermented such as sugar, bread, refined carbohydrates such as white rice and pasta, alcohol, cheese, dried fruit, fruit juices, soy sauce, vinegar, stock cubes and peanuts. At the same time, it is a good idea to take an acidophilus supplement, available from health food stores and pharmacies. This contains bacterial strains to help restore the balance of organisms in the gut. If yeast is the underlying cause of the problem, this dietary regime and acidophilus supplementation should improve symptoms over a two to three month period.

FOOD INTOLERANCE AND IBS

Many sufferers of IBS have their symptoms triggered by certain foods when the gut seems to be unable to cope with the problem food or foods, and this causes reactions which give rise to the symptoms typical of IBS. Just about any food can do this, but by far the most common culprits are milk, cheese and wheat-based foods such as bread, pasta, pastry, pizza, biscuits, cakes, breakfast cereals and crackers. Eliminating these foods can bring about a significant improvement in symptoms in a substantial number of people.

3

KEY FOODS TO AVOID IN IBS

■ Wheat-based products such as bread, pasta, pastry, pizza, wheat crackers, wheat-based breakfast cereals.

■ Breaded food, battered food and foods containing wheat flour.

■ Cow's milk and cheese.

■ Yeasty, mouldy and fermented foods such as yeast-containing bread, stock cubes, gravy mixes, mushrooms, alcohol, soy sauce, vinegar.

■ Sugar and high-sugar foods including biscuits, cakes, chocolate, confectionery, pastries and soft drinks.

■ Peanuts.

■ Dried fruit.

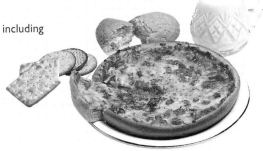

FOODS TO RELIEVE IBS

Although IBS is a complex condition that may involve a number of different factors, including stress, many sufferers have found that eating certain foods can help ease the symptoms of the condition. The two main classes of foods that have been found to be helpful are the high-fibre foods and those that contain healthy gut bacteria. While excluding the foods that tend to make the symptoms of IBS worse (see page 57), increase the amounts of the beneficial foods listed in the box opposite. Because many of these foods are high in vitamins and other nutrients as well as fibre, you are likely to notice that your general health and energy levels are also improved.

FIBRE

A high fibre diet is particularly important in overcoming IBS. Many sufferers turn to high wheat bran cereals as a convenient source of fibre. However, the fibre in such cereals can be too hard on the gut and some sufferers are sensitive to it. Generally, IBS sufferers do much better on foods such as fruit, vegetables and brown rice. If you suffer from IBS, make sure you eat at least five servings of fruit or vegetables each day. Oat-based foods, such as some breakfast cereals and oat cakes, are also good sources of fibre.

3

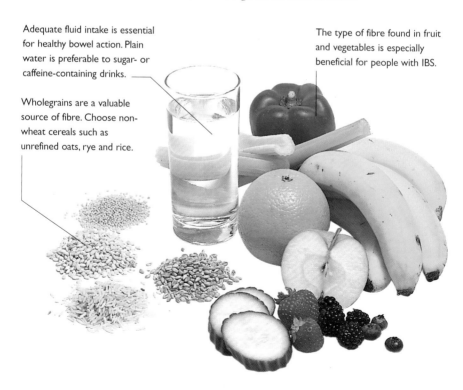

Adequate fluid intake is essential for healthy bowel action. Plain water is preferable to sugar- or caffeine-containing drinks.

Wholegrains are a valuable source of fibre. Choose non-wheat cereals such as unrefined oats, rye and rice.

The type of fibre found in fruit and vegetables is especially beneficial for people with IBS.

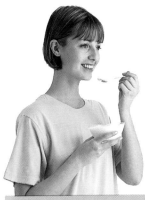

LIVE YOGHURT

The bacterial cultures contained in live yoghurt can have a positive effect on the gut. They can help with digestion and also promote health in the lining of the gut. Eating a pot of natural live yoghurt each day is a good way to keep the level of healthy bacteria in the gut topped up, and many IBS sufferers have found that this can help them to control their symptoms.

STRESS RELIEF AND IBS

Many people who suffer from irritable bowel syndrome notice that their symptoms are worse when they feel stressed or anxious. In conjunction with dietary adjustments, stress reduction and relaxation techniques can be effective in alleviating IBS. Take time each day to practise some form of relaxation such as deep breathing or meditation. Yoga teaches excellent relaxation techniques. Alternatively, many people find regular gentle exercise such as brisk walking both relaxing and helpful for relief of IBS.

3

KEY FOODS TO RELIEVE IBS

The following foods have all been found to be beneficial for IBS sufferers. Some are high in fibre, others are useful substitutes for foods that may aggravate the condition. All the listed foods contain valuable nutrients that will boost your general health.

- Oats and oat products such as porridge, oat muesli and oat cakes.

- Brown rice.

- Yeast-free rye bread and rye crackers.

- Fresh fruit.

- Vegetables.

- Potatoes.

- Water and herb teas (especially peppermint or fennel).

- Nuts (except peanuts).

- Rice milk, soya milk and soya cheese.

- White meat.

- Live natural yoghurt.

- Fish.

- Seafood.

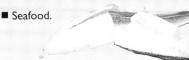

LIVER AND KIDNEYS

The liver and kidneys are the main organs responsible for eliminating waste products and toxins from the blood. These unwanted chemicals may accumulate in the bloodstream as breakdown products from the normal digestion and metabolism of food, or they may be absorbed directly from the gut as in the case of certain drugs or medications. Unless both liver and kidneys are working well, waste products may build up in the bloodstream, leading to serious ill-health.

EATING FOR A HEALTHY LIVER

The liver is the key organ for processing chemicals in the bloodstream – either converting them into a form that the body can use or altering them so that they can be removed by the kidneys. The liver has a particularly important role in the digestion and processing of fat. The health of the liver therefore has an impact on the entire body. Eating or drinking the wrong things can reduce liver efficiency. Drinking too much alcohol and caffeine can stress the liver. Constipation, which can result from a low-fibre, low fluid diet (see page 54), can lead to reabsorption of toxins by the gut which can also overwork the liver. The key dietary considerations for a healthy liver are therefore:

■ Drink plenty of water, to help flush out toxins.

■ Take measures to avoid constipation (see page 54).

■ Keep alcohol and caffeine intake low.

EATING FOR KIDNEY HEALTH

The kidneys are constantly filtering the blood, removing waste chemicals and excess fluid, which then pass out of the body as urine. Except in the case of reduced kidney function, which requires medically monitored dietary measures, what we eat does not have a marked effect on kidney health, although it is important to drink plenty of fluids, preferably water, to keep the system "flushed" and to prevent infection in the urinary tract.

However, some people have a tendency to form "stones" in the kidneys. These are small deposits, usually of calcium oxalate or phosphate. Kidney stones can cause severe pain as they pass through the urinary tract and sufferers usually require medical treatment. If you have a tendency to form oxalate-containing kidney stones, it is often helpful to reduce your intake of foods that are high in oxalic acid, including beetroot, spinach, rhubarb, gooseberries, strawberries, nuts, chocolate and tea.

EATING FOR WEIGHT CONTROL

Obesity is a common problem in the industrialized world and is becoming more common despite growing health consciousness. Besides being a major risk factor for heart disease, obesity can also increase the likelihood of a wide variety of other conditions including diabetes, arthritis and certain forms of cancer. Being overweight or obese can have profound psychological effects, too, and may cause considerable unhappiness.

Crash diets, however, bring their own problems and rarely lead to lasting weight loss.

Instead, excess weight should be lost gradually through sensible, healthy eating.

4

A HEALTHY WEIGHT

To a large degree, a healthy weight is a personal matter. Everyone has a weight and shape that feels most comfortable and, for many people, their ideal weight is better determined on the basis of how they feel rather than from a height and weight table. Although such tables can give a rough guide as to the healthy weight for an individual, they are generally too crude to take account of individual body make-up and characteristics.

OVERWEIGHT OR OBESE?

Overweight and obesity are both conditions in which there is an excess amount of body fat. The difference is merely one of degree, with obesity being the more serious condition. In recent years there has been a tendency to move away from traditional height and weight tables to a form of weight assessment called the body mass index (BMI). You can calculate your BMI precisely by dividing your weight in kilograms by the square of your height in metres. Use this chart to make a quick check on your body mass index. Read across from your height to the point at which you cross the line relating to your weight. The coloured bands indicate broadly if your BMI is healthy.

IS YOUR BODY MASS INDEX HEALTHY?

4

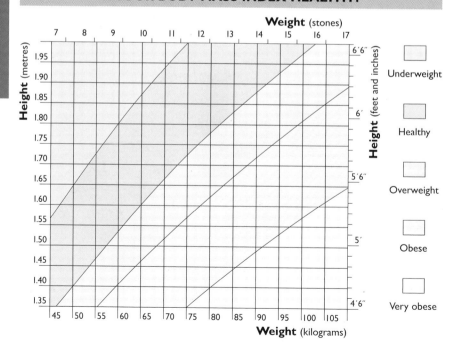

CALCULATING YOUR BODY MASS INDEX

The medically determined bands for the risk of ill-health from a high BMI are slightly different for men and women. If your BMI is borderline according to the chart on the facing page, it is probaby best to do a mathematical calcualtion and check the precise results against the following guidelines.

BMI Men	Band	BMI Women
less than 20	underweight	less than 19
20 – 25	healthy	19 – 24
26 – 30	overweight	25 – 29
31 – 40	obese	30 – 40
more than 41	very obese	more than 41

Underweight

Being underweight is a relatively rare problem and may be associated with chronic illness or an eating disorder such as anorexia nervosa. Those who are underweight may be at increased risk of ill-health.

Healthy

If you fall into this category, your weight is ideal and your aim should be to maintain this level in the coming years.

Overweight

People who fall into this category may have health problems as a result. There is a moderate risk of heart disease at this level of weight and steps should be taken to reduce weight in the long term.

Obese

Obesity is closely associated with ill-health and it is likely that anyone falling into this category will be at significant risk from a wide range of disorders. Steps should be taken to reduce weight immediately.

Very obese

At this weight health is seriously at risk and immediate action to lose weight under medical supervision must be taken.

4

THE PITFALLS OF DIETING

Many weight loss programmes are based on the principle that the fewer calories we eat, the more weight we lose. Although this principle works in most cases in the short term, there are important reasons why the effect cannot be sustained. What is more, long-term calorie restriction can put enormous strain on the body. We now know that severe calorie restriction can have a number of harmful effects and many individuals who diet repeatedly end up hungry, overweight and, paradoxically, malnourished.

THE FLAWED ORIGINS OF THE CALORIE PRINCIPLE

The calorie principle was first put forward in 1930 by two doctors, Newburgh and Johnston, at the University of Michigan, USA. Their original study was conducted over too short a period to draw any conclusion about the long-term effects of calorie restriction, but was nevertheless taken up as the standard approach to weight loss by the medical establishment.

WHY CONVENTIONAL DIETING DOESN'T WORK

Conventional, calorie-controlled dieting may produce dramatic initial falls in weight and fat levels in the body, but also results in muscle loss and a drop in energy levels. Tackling excess weight by using the healthy eating principles outlined in this chapter results in gradual loss of weight and fat, while maintaining muscle bulk and improving energy levels.

4

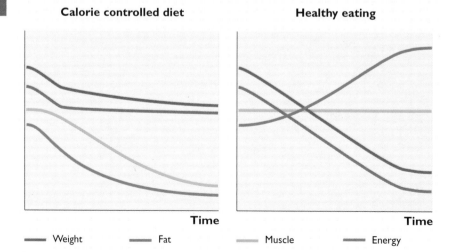

Calorie controlled diet | Healthy eating

Time | Time

▬▬ Weight   ▬▬ Fat   ▬▬ Muscle   ▬▬ Energy

THE EFFECTS OF CALORIE RESTRICTION

Although the calorie principle works initially, the body soon detects that its food intake has been cut and goes into starvation mode, when it does everything it can to preserve the energy stores it has. This means the less you eat in the long term, the less your body will burn – which is why your weight may plateau no matter how little you eat.

WEIGHT LOSS/GAIN CYCLES

Once you abandon a diet and start eating normal volumes of food, the body is suddenly unable to cope with the increased supply and the weight that was lost quickly returns, often with a few pounds added on for good measure. Repeated cycles of weight loss followed by weight gain (weight-cycling) have been shown to have an adverse effect on health, particularly with regard to heart disease.

FAT LOSS OR MUSCLE LOSS?

Losing weight on a strict diet does not mean you are losing fat. In order to make up for the food you are not eating, the body doesn't just break down fat to use as energy, it breaks down protein (muscle) as well. The last thing you need on a diet is to reduce your lean body mass. Conventional diets may lead to weight loss, but body fat percentages often change very little.

FOOD QUALITY

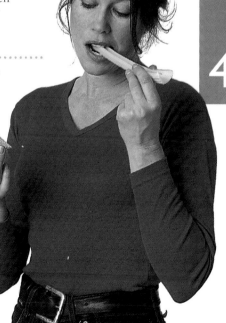

Calorie-based diets place more emphasis on quantity of food rather than the quality. Even an apparently healthy diet is unlikely to supply all the vitamins and minerals we need in the amounts necessary for peak health. When we begin to cut down on the amount of food that we eat, and at the same time eat foods which are low in nutrients (most diet foods are), we are in grave danger of suffering from the effects of vitamin and mineral depletion.

A diet restricted to typical "slimming" foods such as crispbreads and celery cannot meet the body's nutritional needs.

4

MORE MUSCLE, LESS FAT

While the BMI relates overall body weight to height, it is not a reliable measure of body make-up. People who are heavily muscled may have a high BMI, but that doesn't mean they are obese. It's not being overweight that is the problem, it's being over-fat. Ascertaining your body fat percentage (BFP) will help you distinguish between excess fat and a big build.

BODY FAT PERCENTAGE

Body weight is made up of a number of constituents including water, muscle, bone and fat. The parts of the body other than fat make up what is termed the lean body compartment. This makes up between 80 and 85 per cent of body mass in healthy individuals. Body fat is sometimes described as fat mass and, although quite stable in some people, it can be prone to great fluctuations in others. BFPs can be calculated from skin-fold thickness measurements taken with callipers at various sites over the body. Assessments are usually available at sports and leisure facilities and the ideal values for men and women are given in the chart below.

4

BODY FAT PERCENTAGES

This chart shows the percentage of body fat (BFP) that is healthy for both men and women. You will need an expert check from your doctor or fitness adviser to discover what your percentage of body fat is. If you are above the recommended values, the higher your BFP, the greater your risk of all the chronic diseases associated with excess fat such as heart disease, diabetes, high blood pressure, cancer and arthritis. Don't forget that is also possible to have too little body fat.

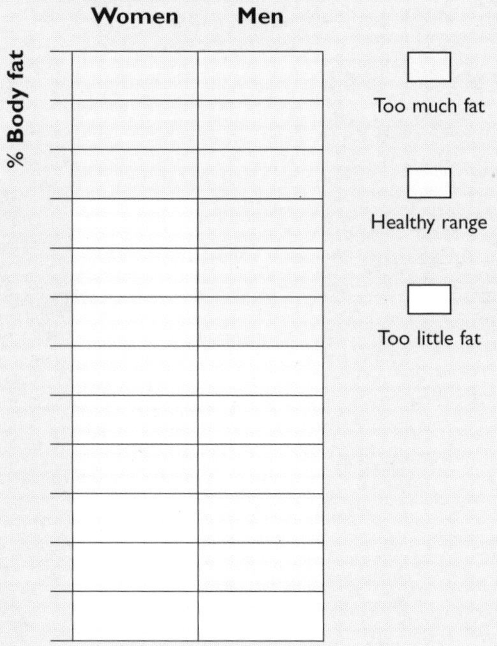

	Women	Men	
% Body fat			☐ Too much fat
			☐ Healthy range
			☐ Too little fat

LOSING FAT, GAINING MUSCLE

It is important to remember that improvements in body composition may lead to little or no change in weight. An individual who is losing fat at a moderate rate is unlikely to see much change in the readings on the scales if he or she is also gaining a degree of muscle through physical exercise. Muscle is actually denser than fat and therefore any increase in the lean muscle mass will often nullify any weight loss that may have been expected through a reduction in fat. However, despite little or no change in actual weight, this change in body composition will have beneficial effects on general health and shape.

SAME WEIGHT, DIFFERENT BODY COMPOSITION

Two people of identical height and weight can have very different body compositions. Because A and B have identical height and weights they also have identical BMIs. However, looking at their body composition we can see that A has a more lean muscle mass. B, on the other hand, has a much higher body fat percentage. Despite having the same weight as A, B quite clearly needs to lose fat and build muscle.

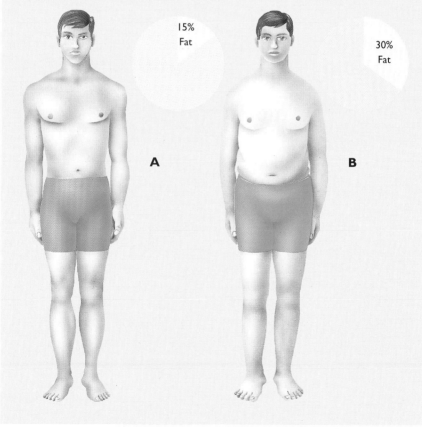

15% Fat

30% Fat

A

B

4

MALE AND FEMALE FAT

Some people find it easier to lose weight than others and one frequent observation is that men generally find it easier to lose weight than women. Men also tend to lose weight from their problem area – the middle – while women find it hard to lose weight from the sites where they tend to accumulate fat – the hips and buttocks. Why? Until now, the reasons for these differences were unknown. However, scientists are now discovering essential differences between male and female fat which have important implications, not only for weight loss, but for general health as well.

WAIST TO HIP RATIOS

The distribution of fat in the body can easily be assessed by making a comparison of the waist circumference to the hip circumference. The so-called waist to hip ratio can help to predict whether excess body fat is likely to be putting us at risk of illness. For women the waist measurement should be no more than 85 per cent of that of the hips. For men the figure is 95 per cent. By plotting your waist and hip measurements on the chart below, you can discover whether your hip to waist ratio is within the healthy range. If your measurements fall into the "unhealthy" area, you may be at greater risk from health problems such as reduced HDL (good) cholesterol, high blood pressure, high total cholesterol and diabetes later in life.

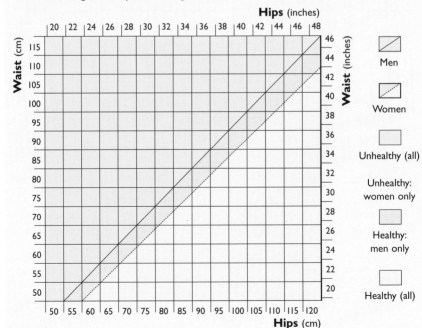

MALE FAT

The differences between male and female fat seem to be related to their distribution. The fat that men store around the chest and stomach – known as abdominal fat – is surplus to requirements, and the body is therefore more than happy to lose it so most men tend to lose weight relatively easily.

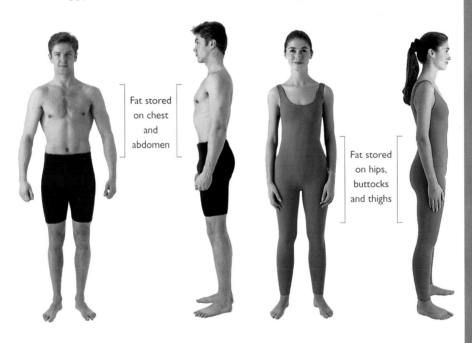

Fat stored on chest and abdomen

Fat stored on hips, buttocks and thighs

4

FEMALE FAT

The fat that women store around the hips, upper thighs and buttocks – known as gluteal fat – appears to have an important function as an energy reserve in pregnancy and during breast-feeding. Because of this essential role in reproduction, gluteal fat is resistant to dieting, and this is why so many women find it so difficult to shift. Women who have struggled to lose weight in the past may take comfort from the knowledge that the reason for this is simply a natural part of womanhood and not a personal failing.

FAT DISTRIBUTION AND HEALTH

Fat distribution not only seems to determine speed of weight loss, but also its effect on health. Obesity has long been known to increase the risk of a number of major illnesses and premature death. Interestingly, it appears that abdominal fat is the significant risk factor here, while gluteal fat is thought to have little or no harmful effect on health. So, although men may find it easier to lose weight than women, the risks they face by remaining overweight are considerably greater.

FOOD INTOLERANCE

Adverse reactions to food are an important cause of weight gain in some individuals. The immune system is programmed to react to anything that appears foreign in the body such as bacteria and viruses. However, it will also tend to react to incompletely digested food.

THE IMMUNE RESPONSE AND WEIGHT GAIN

It is thought that in some people, particles of undigested or partially digested food leak through the intestinal wall into the bloodstream, and come in contact with the immune system, triggering a reaction. One of the effects of this immune reaction is fluid retention in the body, leading to weight gain. The foods that cause problems vary from person to person. Some people are sensitive to the proteins in cow's milk and products derived from cow's milk, whereas others may react to wheat or citrus fruits.

COMMON FOODS THAT CREATE INTOLERANCE

A number of common foods can trigger sensitivity in susceptible individuals. Wheat and foods containing wheat flour are among the most frequently found causes of food intolerance. Citrus fruit and cow's milk are also responsible for food sensitivity in a large number of people.

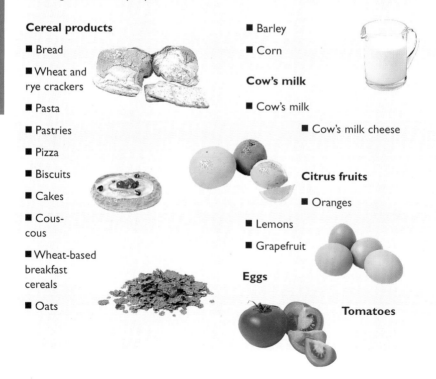

Cereal products

- Bread
- Wheat and rye crackers
- Pasta
- Pastries
- Pizza
- Biscuits
- Cakes
- Couscous
- Wheat-based breakfast cereals
- Oats

- Barley
- Corn

Cow's milk

- Cow's milk
- Cow's milk cheese

Citrus fruits

- Oranges
- Lemons
- Grapefruit

Eggs

Tomatoes

4

WHAT CAUSES FOOD INTOLERANCE?

There are many factors that may contribute to the development of food intolerance. Many food intolerances start early in life. Quite often foods are introduced into a child's diet when the intestinal tract and immune system are relatively immature and, as a result, the child is unable to deal appropriately with the food, causing a sensitivity to it. Infants who are bottle fed, for instance, often become sensitive to cow's milk formula feeds. This can manifest in a number of ways but colic and eczema are common signs. Breast-fed infants are less likely to develop food intolerance.

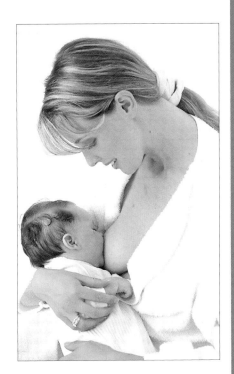

Breastfeeding is one of the best ways of preventing your child developing food intolerance.

CHANGES IN OUR FOOD

There is a theory that food intolerances are becoming more common because we are eating more and more foods that are relatively recent additions to our diet and we just have not had long enough to adjust to these new foods. For example, although we have cultivated and eaten wheat for many thousands of years, the form of wheat we eat now is quite different from the form of wheat on which we evolved. Milk is another example. Although we have drunk milk for quite some time during our evolution, it was predominantly goat's and sheep's milk, not milk from cows.

4

IMMUNE REACTIONS

The immune reactions caused by food intolerance are thought to be at the root of a wide range of conditions including eczema, sinusitis, migraine, rheumatoid arthritis and weight gain. Many individuals find that identifying and eliminating problem foods from the diet can lead to significant weight loss and an improvement in overall health.

POOR DIGESTION

Other theories about the cause of food intolerance revolve around poor digestion and a gut which tends to leak particles into the bloodstream. Poor chewing and/or a lack of stomach acid or digestive enzymes may cause poor digestion, while an imbalance in the organisms in the gut and other factors such as toxins in the diet may contribute to a leaky gut.

IS THIS MY PROBLEM?

There are certain symptoms or signs which are clues to whether food intolerance is likely to be a problem for you. Some of these you may be able to recognize yourself. If your symptoms suggest that you may be suffering from food intolerance, the next step is to identify the particular food that may be the cause of the problem. In some cases it may be obvious which food is the culprit, but if you are unsure there are several methods used by "alternative" practitioners to test for specific food sensitivities.

KEY QUESTIONS

By answering the following questions you can determine whether food intolerance is likely to be a factor in your health.

■ Do you suffer from fluid retention from time to time (classic signs are puffy ankles, hands and fingers and fluctuations in weight by a few pounds from day to day)?

■ Do you feel lethargic soon after eating?

■ Do you feel better when you don't eat?

■ Did you have reactions to foods when you were younger?

■ Do you have recurrent, unexplained symptoms?

■ Do you have dark circles under your eyes?

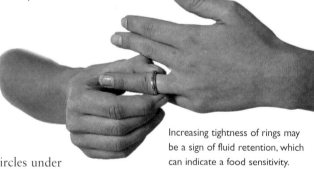

Increasing tightness of rings may be a sign of fluid retention, which can indicate a food sensitivity.

If you answered yes to most of these questions, then it is likely that you are intolerant to one or more foods. In this case dealing with the food intolerance can lead to improved long-term weight control.

THE ELIMINATION DIET

An elimination diet involves cutting out all foods that are likely to cause a problem for about three weeks. If an improvement is detected, then foods can be added back into the diet, one every day or two. Foods that cause a recurrence of the original symptoms are then identified as the problem foods. This method of testing is generally believed to be quite accurate, though it is time consuming and laborious.

4

BLOOD TESTING FOR FOOD INTOLERANCE

There are several blood tests that diagnose food intolerance. One test, the cytotoxic test, is undertaken by mixing immune cells with individual food extracts to ascertain which food extracts cause reactions in the immune cells. Another test measures antibodies in the blood to specific foods. The accuracy of some blood tests have been called into question and they also tend to be quite expensive.

ELECTRO-DERMAL TESTING

Also known as Vega testing, this method involves measuring the electrical current that flows through the body and then detecting any changes in it as the body is challenged with individual foods. In skilled hands this method seems to give good and instantaneous results. Electro-dermal testing is relatively cheap compared to blood tests.

APPLIED KINESIOLOGY

This is similar to electro-dermal testing except that the practitioner measures muscle strength in response to foods rather than electrical current. Like electro-dermal testing, the results are thought to be relatively accurate in skilled hands and the results are instantaneous. Again, testing tends to be inexpensive compared to blood tests for food intolerance.

CONSULTING A PRACTITIONER

In order to pinpoint the foods to which you may be intolerant, it is often helpful to consult a qualified nutritionist or natural health practitioner. As well as helping you to identify possible problem foods in your case, he or she will be able to give advice on a sensible and safe diet that willl ensure that you receive adequate and balanced nutrition. Always seek expert advice before adopting a diet that excludes a large number of foods that have formed part of your regular diet. A reputable practitioner will always ask for a detailed medical history in order to exclude the possibility of an underlying condition that requires medical treatment.

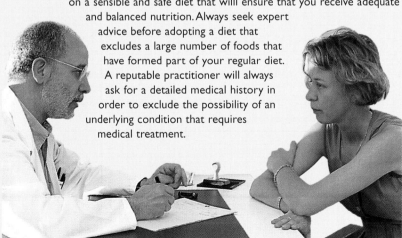

4

BLOOD SUGAR AND WEIGHT

One very important factor in ensuring healthy weight loss is maintaining a stable level of sugar in the bloodstream. When food is eaten, the level of sugar in the bloodstream rises. The pancreas responds to this by secreting a hormone called insulin. Insulin facilitates the absorption of sugar into the body's cells, and this process is essential to the regulation of the blood sugar level.

HOW HIGH BLOOD SUGAR CAUSES WEIGHT GAIN

Some foods cause the blood sugar level to rise rapidly. (These are discussed more fully on pages 12–15.) In response to the sudden presence of high levels of sugar in the blood, insulin is released, which converts the sugar that is not required for instant use as energy into fat for storage in the tissues. So eating foods that release sugar quickly will tend to cause weight gain over a prolonged period.

HIGHS AND LOWS

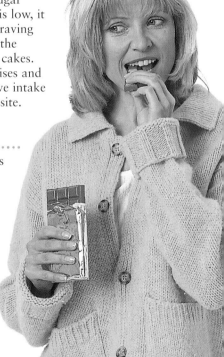

The body acts quickly to compensate for rapid rises in blood sugar. The processes that are designed to keep levels of sugar in the blood within healthy limits tend to over-react, which can lead to low blood sugar some time later. When the blood sugar level is low, it is natural for the appetite to be stimulated, craving foods that tend to release sugar quickly into the bloodstream, such as chocolate, biscuits and cakes. This initiates a damaging cycle of dramatic rises and falls in blood sugar levels along with excessive intake of sugary foods, as shown in the graph opposite.

4

FATIGUE

A natural downside to low blood sugar levels is fatigue, leading many individuals to avoid exercise. Regular exercise is essential for the maintenance of energy levels and optimum body function. Lack of exercise is, of course, an important contributing factor in excess weight gain.

Eating something sweet such as chocolate is likely to make symptoms of low blood sugar worse in the long term.

LOSING WEIGHT THROUGH BLOOD SUGAR CONTROL

Eating the right diet can help stabilize the blood sugar level and so help to bring about weight loss. Remember the following guidelines:

- Do not skip meals.

- Eat regular small meals rather than less frequent large meals.

- Base your diet around low glycaemic index foods that release sugar slowly into the bloodstream.

- Avoid foods that raise blood sugar excessively.

GLYCAEMIC INDEX

The rate at which sugar is released into the bloodstream can be quantified using a measure called the glycaemic index. Foods that are absorbed rapidly have a high glycaemic index, while foods which are more slowly absorbed have a low glycaemic index (see pages 12–15). Generally, sugars have higher glycaemic indices than starches. However, some starchy foods such as potatoes and refined carbohydrates, such as white bread, white rice and pasta, have high glycaemic indices and should be eaten in moderation.

Anyone wishing to stabilize their blood sugar levels should base their diet around foods of low glycaemic index, such as meat, fish, unrefined wholegrains (wholemeal bread, brown rice, wholewheat pasta), beans, pulses, fruit and vegetables.

BLOOD SUGAR LEVELS AFTER EATING

This chart compares the blood sugar levels after eating a high glycaemic index food, such as chocolate, and after eating a low glycaemic index food such as fruit.

4

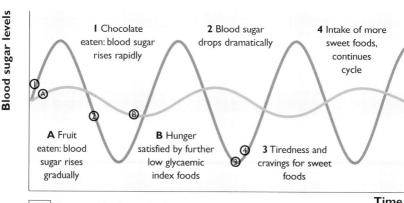

I Chocolate eaten: blood sugar rises rapidly

2 Blood sugar drops dramatically

4 Intake of more sweet foods, continues cycle

A Fruit eaten: blood sugar rises gradually

B Hunger satisfied by further low glycaemic index foods

3 Tiredness and cravings for sweet foods

Optimum blood sugar level

Time

Blood sugar levels

FOOD MYTHS

The food industry offers an array of foods targeted towards the weight-conscious public. Low-fat or low-sugar versions of many foods are found on supermarket shelves. However, the value of these foods as aids to slimming is debatable, and some of these foods provide poorer nutritional value than their "fattening" equivalents.

LOW-FAT FOODS

Supermarket shelves are packed with products declaring themselves to be low in fat, "lite", or cholesterol free. The question is, are they really any more healthy than their full-fat versions? More important than the percentage of fat in a food is the percentage of the calories contributed by fat. To calculate this we have to multiply the number of grams of fat in a food by nine, divide this by the total number of calories and multiply by 100. Using this calculation we can see many foods that claim to be low in fat are actually very fatty. For example, regular cream cheese is 30 per cent fat and has 86 per cent of its calories coming from fat. Low-fat cream cheese has 15 per cent fat, half the amount of fat of the full-fat version. However, doing the sums reveals that the percentage of calories coming from fat is 73, which is not a significant "saving". Many low-fat foods, such as low-fat ice-cream, biscuits or yoghurt, also have extra sugar and starch added to maintain palatability and texture. For health and weight control it is simpler to cut down on high-fat foods and substitute increased amounts of healthy foods such as fresh fruit and vegetables.

4

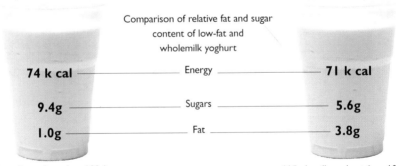

Comparison of relative fat and sugar
content of low-fat and
wholemilk yoghurt

74 k cal	Energy	71 k cal
9.4g	Sugars	5.6g
1.0g	Fat	3.8g

Low-fat yoghurt (per 100g)   Wholemilk yoghurt (per 100g)

ARTIFICIAL SWEETENERS

Along with fat, the other major food component that we have been encouraged to cut back on is sugar. Many foodstuffs now have some or all of the sugar content replaced with artificial sweeteners such as aspartame and saccharin. However, there is some scientific evidence to suggest that artificial sweeteners may actually encourage us to eat more in the long term. In one study, people were inclined to eat more after eating yoghurt sweetened with saccharin than those who had eaten yoghurt sweetened with sugar.

DIET DRINKS

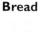

Apart from artificial sweeteners, another potential health hazard in many diet drinks is caffeine. Caffeine produces a temporary feeling of energy, alertness and well-being. The problem is that it is also addictive, and many of us depend on it to give us that jolt we need to get us through the day. Regular caffeine consumption can quite easily lead to fatigue, headache, depression, insomnia, irritability and anxiety. There are also serious questions over the role caffeine has to play in the development of cancer of the prostate, pancreas and bladder.

"SLIMMING" FOODS

Although diet foods and drinks are promoted as a blessing for the would-be slimmer, the fact is their advertised benefits are often more the result of marketing hype than nutritional fact. The claim made by the manufacturers of many of these diet products is that they can help you lose weight only as part of a calorie-controlled diet. The truth is that any food, however many calories or unhealthy ingredients it contains, can "help" weight loss when eaten in conjunction with a calorie-controlled diet. It is the calorie restriction, not the food, that leads to the weight loss. What is more, weight-for-weight, many slimming food products contain nearly as many calories as non-slimming equivalents. The only reason that some products are able to boast fewer calories per portion is that the size of the serving is smaller than that of the regular product.

4

COMPARING SLIMMING AND NORMAL FOODS

Food	Normal	Slimming
Soup (dried)	(per 100g) Calories 380 kcal Protein 7g Carbohydrate 68g of which sugar 18g Fat 9g Portion size 24g	(per 100g) Calories 315 kcal Protein 11g Carbohydrate 60g of which sugar 25g Fat 4g Portion size 15g
Bread	Calories 210 kcal Protein 10g Carbohydrate 38g of which sugar 3g Fat 2g Portion size 44g	Calories 235 kcal Protein 8g Carbohydrate 46g of which sugar 4g Fat 2g Portion size 21g

LASTING WEIGHT LOSS

If you are planning to lose weight, the best way to achieve this is undoubtedly through a sensible and healthy approach to your diet. The key is to make lasting changes to your eating habits. This should not involve a phase of semi-starvation that leaves you craving sweets and pastries, but should be focused on improving the overall balance of your diet. Using the analogy of the body as a furnace, the fire represents our metabolism, and the fuel is the food we eat. In order to keep the furnace burning we need to ensure that we use the right fuel and put it on the fire on a regular basis.

QUALITY FOODS

In simple terms healthy eating means eating good quality food according to a sensible pattern. Junk foods such as fast foods, sweets, cakes and confectionery are a bit like damp logs on the fire – they don't burn very well. Fruit, vegetables and wholegrains such as wholemeal bread burn much better. A good approach is to focus on the nutritional value of any food you eat in addition to the energy it provides. Pure sugar provides only empty calories in that it has no additional nutrients, whereas fruit, for example, provides essential vitamins and fibre as well as natural sugars. Try to eat only foods that have a positive nutritional benefit.

FOOD AS FUEL

Some dieters think that skipping meals and going hungry must be the best way to lose weight, though by comparing this idea to the furnace analogy, it is plain how mistaken this is. If we light a fire at breakfast time and don't fuel it in the middle of the day, what happens by the time we come back to the fire in the evening? The flame will be so low that the fuel we put on it in the evening will not burn easily at all. Skipped meals mean, in fact, that the body is more likely to store subsequent meals as fat.

Do not think that because you want to lose weight, you have to eat less; you simply need to eat differently. It is quite likely that you will benefit from eating more frequently than you have been used to to avoid the distorted food cravings caused by low blood sugar (see page 74). But remember to choose all the food you eat carefully, for maximum nutritional benefit.

4

TEN-POINT PLAN FOR WEIGHT CONTROL

This ten-point guide to healthy eating covers the basics of healthy nutrition that will also ensure weight loss.

1 Eat three meals a day

Regular meals are important if the metabolism is to be properly fed and they also help to ensure that blood sugar levels are maintained, preventing hunger and food cravings.

2 Eat a healthy snack if you get hungry between meals

Eating something healthy between meals can also help to keep blood sugar levels stable during the day. Fresh and dried fruit, raw vegetables, nuts and seeds make ideal snacks.

3 Drink healthily

Avoid caffeine as it stimulates your body to secrete insulin and this can lower blood sugar. Soft drinks are full of sugar and/or artificial chemical additives and are best avoided. The healthiest drinks are still mineral water and freshly squeezed fruit and vegetable juices.

4 Drink alcohol only in moderation

A small amount of alcohol is compatible with a healthy diet but larger amounts can be very fattening. Aim to drink no more than one or two units of alcohol per day.

5 Drink mainly between meals and not at mealtimes

Drinking at mealtimes dilutes the secretions which digest food and therefore disturbs the digestion. Poor digestion is often a factor in weight gain.

6 Cut down on fat

When choosing protein-rich foods, choose fish rather than meat. Poultry (without the skin) is generally healthier than red meats such as beef, lamb and pork. When eating dairy products, go for the low-fat varieties wherever possible such as low-fat cheese, skimmed or semi-skimmed milk and low-fat (unsweetened) yoghurt.

continued ▶

▶ *continued*

TEN-POINT PLAN FOR WEIGHT CONTOL

7 Identify and eliminate your food sensitivities

Finding out which foods your body tends to be sensitive to and eliminating them from your diet can bring about a very significant weight loss in susceptible individuals. Common culprits are wheat and dairy products.

8 Choose unrefined carbohydrates

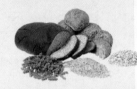

These foods contain far more in the way of fibre, vitamins and minerals than their more refined and processed versions. They also release sugar relatively slowly into the bloodstream and this helps maintain blood sugar stability. Examples of unrefined carbohydrates include wholemeal or other 100 per cent wholegrain bread, brown rice, potatoes in their jackets and wholewheat pasta.

9 Avoid sugar

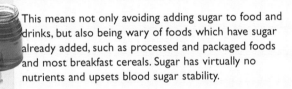

This means not only avoiding adding sugar to food and drinks, but also being wary of foods which have sugar already added, such as processed and packaged foods and most breakfast cereals. Sugar has virtually no nutrients and upsets blood sugar stability.

10 Eat plenty of fresh fruit and vegetables

High in nutrients and fibre, these foods are an essential part of any healthy diet. Aim to eat five servings of fresh fruit or vegetables every day (one serving is a piece of fruit such as an apple or banana or a helping of salad or vegetables). Vegetables are better either raw (such as a salad), steamed or microwaved. These forms of food preparation preserve more of the nutrients in the food than boiling, baking or frying.

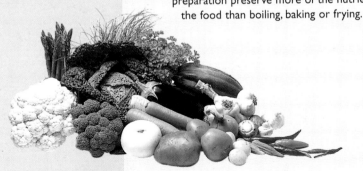

4

EATING FOR IMMUNE HEALTH

A healthy immune system protects us from potentially harmful bacteria and viruses. If it is weakened, infections such as colds and flu are more likely. Another major role for the immune system is in the prevention of cancer. It is constantly detecting and destroying abnormal cells, which if unchecked could develop into cancer. Therefore weakness of the immune system can increase our risk of cancer. Illness can also sometimes be due to overactivity of the immune system – as occurs, for instance, in rheumatoid arthritis. The latest research shows that both underactivity and overactivity of the immune system can be improved by eating the right kind of diet.

5

THE IMMUNE SYSTEM

The immune system is made up of a number of different types of cells, known collectively as "white blood cells". The most important of these are the B- and T-cells. The B-cells produce antibodies, special proteins that help keep viruses out of the body's cells and assist in the neutralization of bacteria. T-cells come in a number of different forms, the most important of which is the T-helper cell. Helper cells are responsible for deciding on the tactics for the whole of the immune defence system and for instructing the B-cells to make antibodies.

B AND T CELLS

B- and T-cells are to be found mainly in the bloodstream and the lymphatic system. Within the immune system are areas where immune cells tend to be concentrated, called the lymph nodes. These can be found all over the body but can sometimes be felt in certain sites such as the neck, groin and armpit. Should an infection take hold in the body, B- and T-cells will activate and multiply – which is why the "glands" in the neck can enlarge and feel tender during an infection.

CANCER CELLS

Another function of the immune system is to seek and destroy cancer cells. Cancerous cells are, in fact, continually being formed in the body, but a healthy immune system ensures that these cells do not develop into tumours. A weakened immune system, however, may not be able to detect or destroy cancerous cells efficiently and this may increase risk of a cancer developing in the long term.

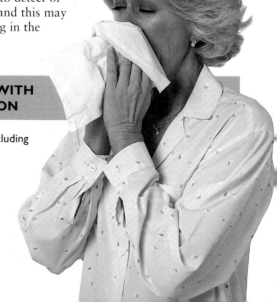

PROBLEMS ASSOCIATED WITH LOW IMMUNE FUNCTION

■ Susceptibility to viral infections including colds, flu and cold sores.

■ Fatigue and chronic fatigue (ME).

■ Cancer.

■ Allergies such as hay fever and asthma.

FRIEND OR FOE?

The immune system is programmed to react to anything that may threaten the body – such as bacteria, viruses, parasites and cancer cells. It is thought that, while we are in the womb, the immune system learns to recognize the body's tissues as a normal part of its environment, differentiating between its own organs and external threats.

AUTO-IMMUNE DISEASE

In some instances, this mechanism by which the body recognizes invaders breaks down and can lead to the development of a condition known as "auto-immune disease". Some auto-immune diseases involve only a specific body organ. One example of a specific auto-immune disease is childhood diabetes, where the immune system reacts to the cells in the pancreas responsible for making insulin. Other auto-immune diseases are more generalized and many parts of the body may be affected. An example of a more non-specific auto-immune disease is rheumatoid arthritis, caused by the immune system's reaction to tissues in several sites around the body.

AUTO-IMMUNE DISEASES

Disease name	Affected organ	Effects of disease
Addison's disease	Adrenal glands	Extreme muscle weakness, low blood pressure, confusion, coma
Auto-immune infertility	Testis or ovary	Infertility
Childhood diabetes	Pancreas	Thirst, increased urination, fatigue, weight loss
Graves' disease	Thyroid	Enlarged thyroid gland (goitre), anxiety, insomnia
Pernicious anaemia	Stomach lining	Fatigue, breathlessness, weight loss, sore mouth
Vitiligo	Skin	Patchy loss of pigment in the skin
Rheumatoid arthritis	Joints	Swelling, redness and pain in the joints, general malaise
Systemic lupus erythematosus (SLE)	Connective tissue	Rash, fatigue, weight loss, joint pain, kidney and heart problems

5

DIET AND IMMUNE HEALTH

The efficiency of the immune system is to some degree dependent on the fuel we give it. Certain foods contain nutrients which are known to have quite potent immune-stimulating effects, which can be used to improve resistance to infection and to help in the fight against cancer. In some people certain foods may trigger an inappropriate immune response, a condition called food sensitivity.

FOOD SENSITIVITY AND THE IMMUNE RESPONSE

Excessive reactions to food by the immune system can be broadly divided into two separate conditions: food allergy and food intolerance. Food allergy – in which sufferers usually experience an obvious reaction to a particular food soon after eating it – is relatively uncommon. In some cases the result is harmless, such as the rash some individuals suffer after eating strawberries. In severe cases, food allergy can produce life-threatening anaphylactic shock, but food allergy sufferers usually find it quite easy to pinpoint the culprit food and then to avoid it.

SYMPTOMS OF FOOD INTOLERANCE

Food intolerance is quite different from food allergy and much more common. With food intolerance, symptoms may develop several hours or even days after eating the culprit food and can be very vague or generalized. Because of this delayed and non-specific reaction, food intolerance often goes undiagnosed, and some people may suffer unnecessarily for many years. Premenstrual syndrome, weight gain, fluid retention, migraine, fatigue, asthma, eczema, irritable bowel syndrome, rheumatoid arthritis and hyperactivity in children are just some of the conditions that have been linked to food intolerance. (See also pages 70–71.)

The likelihood of food intolerance can be minimized by careful attention to diet from babyhood onwards.

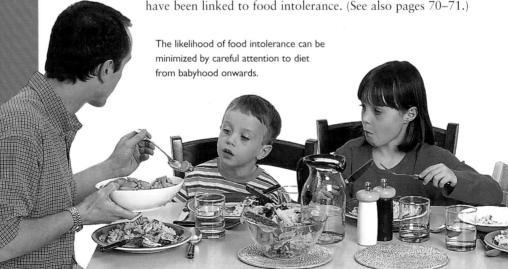

IMMUNE-BOOSTING NUTRIENTS

The following nutrients play a key role in boosting healthy immune function:

Vitamin C

More than a dozen immune-stimulating roles for vitamin C have been identified to date including the ability to increase antibody production and speed the rate at which immune cells mature. Vitamin C is found in highest concentration in bananas, citrus fruits, kiwi fruit and green vegetables.

Zinc

Zinc is critical for the production and function of immune cells and scientific studies have demonstrated that low levels of zinc in the body can lead to a weakening of the immune system. Zinc is found most plentifully in seafood, fish and wholegrains such as wholemeal bread.

Beta-carotene

Beta-carotene is converted into vitamin A in the body. It helps protect the immune system from the action of damaging free radical molecules and also appears to have powerful immune-enhancing properties. Foods rich in beta-carotene include green and yellow fruit and vegetables.

MEAL SIZE

There is a direct correlation between the amount of food the body has to deal with in the system and the efficiency of the immune system. The more we eat, the more incapacitated our immune system becomes. For the best immune function, it makes sense to avoid large meals – in particular, heavy, fatty foods such as red meat and dairy products should be avoided.

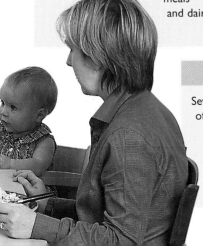

SUGAR AND IMMUNE HEALTH

5

Several scientific studies have shown that, as the level of sugar in the bloodstream goes up, the efficiency of the immune system comes down. All forms of refined sugar have this effect, so keep your diet as low in sugar, sweets, biscuits and soft drinks as possible.

THE CAUSES OF CANCER

The body is composed of trillions of cells and, in most tissues, these are gradually but constantly renewed. This is normally a controlled process, so that overall, just enough new cells are produced to replace the old, dead ones. Problems can occur when new, abnormal cells are formed whose multiplication cannot be controlled by the body.

WHAT IS CANCER?

Usually, the body's immune system rapidly destroys any abnormal cells. Cancer comes about when an abnormal cell, unchecked by the immune system, begins to multiply uncontrolledly. When a group of abnormal cells is produced, in time a tumour can form. Tumours that are cancerous are often described as "malignant" and they have a tendency to spread, not only locally, but also to distant parts of the body. A cancer that has spread from an original site is known as a metastasis or secondary, the original being referred to as the primary. In the industrialized world, one in three people will develop cancer at some point in their lives, and one in every four people will die from the disease.

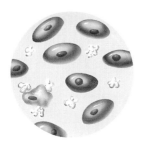
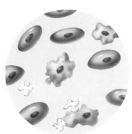
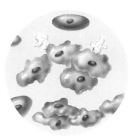

Healthy immune activity
White blood cells attack and destroy abnormal cancer cells.

Lowered immunity
Lack of white blood cells allows the number of cancer cells to increase.

Tumour formation
Eventually the increasing numbers of cancer cells may accumulate to form a tumour.

5

WHAT CAUSES CANCER?

Because cancer is actually a collection of different diseases, there are a large number of potential causes, and risk factors for one type of cancer may not be the same for another. Smoking, for example, is the main risk factor in lung cancer, but not skin cancer. At the heart of the cancer-causing process are destructive substances, generated when the body's cells use oxygen to burn food for energy. This process of combustion can lead to the production of free radical molecules that can, in turn, damage cells, setting off undesirable biochemical reactions which may trigger cancer.

MEDICAL TREATMENT

Malignant tumours, if left without treatment, almost invariably prove fatal. Treatment is usually in the form of drug therapy (chemotherapy), radiotherapy, surgery or a combination of the three. The aim of surgery is usually to stop the cancer from spreading. Some cancers are more easily cured than others. What is almost universally true is that, the earlier the cancer is diagnosed, the better the outlook and the better the prospects of a full recovery.

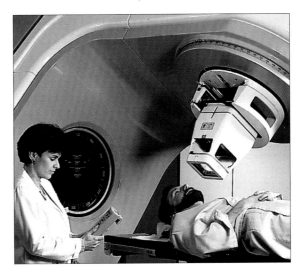

Modern screening methods help doctors to diagnose cancer early, thereby improving the chances of successful treatment.

MALIGNANT AND BENIGN TUMOURS

Not all tumours are malignant – that is, cancerous. Many are not aggressive and, even though they can grow quite large, they do not tend to invade local tissues or spread to other parts of the body. Such tumours are described as benign. Benign tumours are generally harmless and do not usually recur once they have been removed surgically.

THE ROLE OF ANTI-OXIDANTS IN CANCER

Anti-oxidant nutrients such as the vitamins A, C, E and the mineral selenium (see page 91) protect against cancer because they interfere with the very processes that trigger cancer, and at the same time stimulate the immune system to destroy cancer cells before they get into their stride. Essentially, the more anti-oxidants there are present in our body, the less chance there is of our getting cancer. So reducing our risk of cancer is really a matter of keeping our anti-oxidant defences in good shape.

5

While there is no unequivocal evidence that alterations in diet can alter the progress of the disease once it has become established, it makes sense for anyone suffering from cancer to boost their intake of anti-oxidants to give their body the help it needs in its fight against the disease. A healthy vitamin-rich diet forms a vital part of the care offered by specialist cancer units.

CANCER AND DIET

Experts who study the causes of cancer believe that a large number of cancer deaths could be prevented by making sensible changes to our diet. In fact, many scientists believe that up to 70 per cent of all cancers are caused by diet-related factors.

DIETARY FAT AND CANCER

The amount of fat in the diet is linked with an increased risk of cancer, particularly to cancers of the breast, lung, colon, rectum, ovary and prostate. The precise role of fat in cancer is not yet known, although some evidence exists to suggest that high levels of fats in the blood are important for the growth of certain tumours.

FREE RADICALS

Another possible mechanism to explain the link between fat and cancer relates to the action of substances called free radicals (see also page 22). It appears that fats obtained from our diet are particularly susceptible to the action of free radicals and may be converted into forms called trans fats (see below) by free radicals. These altered fats may play an important role in the triggering of cancerous changes in body cells. Anti-oxidants (page 23) from the diet neutralize the action of free radicals and fats in the body. So, the greater the ratio of fat and oils to anti-oxidants in the body, the greater seems the risk of developing cancer.

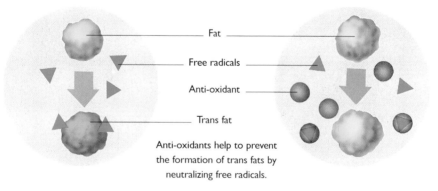

Fat

Free radicals

Anti-oxidant

Trans fat

Anti-oxidants help to prevent
the formation of trans fats by
neutralizing free radicals.

TRANS FATS IN THE DIET

There is evidence that the high temperatures used in the manufacture of margarine and many vegetable oils, and in the preparation of many processed and pre-packaged foods, changes the chemical structure of the fat they contain. These altered fats are known as trans fatty acids (trans fats or TFAs). The body cannot deal with these fats as easily as with the natural fats, and there is some suspicion that TFAs may be a cause of disease, including cancer.

SALT-CURED, SALT-PICKLED, SMOKED FOODS AND CANCER

Eating large amounts of salt-cured, salt-pickled and smoked foods has been linked to cancer of the

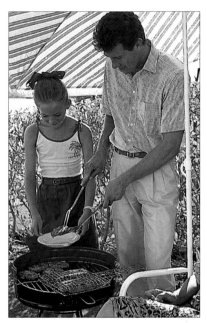

oesophagus. The smoke from curing seems to create cancer-causing substances (carcinogens) in the food, while salt-cured and salt-pickled foods contain chemicals that can be converted into carcinogens in the food or in the stomach.

BARBECUED FOOD

Grilling or barbecuing food over an open flame can also create carcinogens on the surface of foods, particularly if the food is charred and fatty. Obviously, the occasional barbecue meal is unlikely to create a serious cancer risk. But if char-grilled meats form a regular part of your diet, it may be sensible to consider cutting down on these foods.

ALCOHOL AND CANCER

The consumption of alcohol appears to increase the risk of developing certain forms of cancer. In moderate amounts, alcohol seems to be linked to an increased risk of cancers of the breast, rectum and pancreas. In excessive amounts, especially when combined with cigarette smoking, alcohol may also increase the likelihood of cancer of the mouth, oesophagus and larynx. Very heavy drinkers who have cirrhosis of the liver are more prone to liver cancer, too.

To a degree, the link between cancer and alcohol is confused by the fact that individuals who drink quite a lot of alcohol are more likely to smoke and have poor diets. How much is due to the alcohol itself and how much is due to these other factors is in doubt. However, there is emerging evidence about the correlation between moderate consumption of alcohol and an overall improvement in life expectancy (see pages 40–41).

ANTI-CANCER FOODS

Because cancers are very varied and the causes of the disease are complex – and so far not fully understood – there can be no firm guarantee that dietary measures can prevent cancer. However, just as some foods may increase the risk of cancers, there are others that may actually help protect against them.

FRUIT, VEGETABLES AND WHOLEGRAINS

Increasing the amount of fresh fruit, vegetables and wholegrain cereals we eat is the key dietary measure that may help protect us from cancer. These foods contain an abundance of fibre, vitamins and minerals, which have been shown to have a protective effect against the development of a number of different cancers. The relative decline in the intake of these foods in the industrialized world in favour of high-fat and high-sugar processed foods may in part explain the increase in certain forms of cancer.

THE FUNCTION OF FIBRE

Fibre, the part of plant foods which humans cannot completely digest or absorb, is vital to the health of the digestive tract (see also Chapter 3, Eating for Digestive Health). In particular, eating adequate amounts of fibre reduces our risk of colonic cancer. Some scientists believe that certain foods contain toxins or chemicals that may induce cancerous changes in the lining of the colon. It is thought that by speeding the passage of food through the intestine, fibre reduces the time during which these chemicals can have this effect.

OBESITY AND CANCER

Women who are overweight or obese appear to be at increased risk of cancers of the breast and uterus (womb). Studies also suggest that obese men may have increased likelihood of cancers of the prostate and colon. The reason for these findings is not entirely clear, though they may have something to do with dietary factors such as fat and fibre consumption. A healthy body weight therefore seems to be important in reducing the risk of cancer. See also Chapter 4, Eating for Weight Control.

ANTI-CANCER ACTION PLAN

The World Cancer Research Fund guidelines designed to lower cancer risk are:

- Cut down on the amount of fat in the diet. The proportion of energy in the diet derived from fat should be under 30 per cent.

- Increase intake of fruit, vegetables and wholegrain cereals.

- Reduce intake of salt-cured, salt-pickled and smoked foods.

- Drink alcohol in moderation, if at all.

5

KEY ANTI-CANCER NUTRIENTS

Vitamins and minerals play an important role in the fight against cancer, too. Many of these nutrients have anti-oxidant properties, helping to control the free radicals implicated in cancer. Some of the nutrients which are thought to be of particular value are indicated in the chart below.

NUTRIENT	BENEFITS	FOOD SOURCES
Beta-carotene	Converted to vitamin A by the body, and is thought to protect against several cancers, particularly cancer of the lung.	Abundant in fruits and vegetables that are deep yellow or orange in colour, such as red and yellow peppers, carrots, sweet potatoes, peaches, apricots and bananas.
Vitamin A	Protects against several cancers, but it can be toxic, and excessive intake should be avoided pariularly in pregnancy or when planning pregnancy. Supplements should be taken only under medical supervision.	As for beta-carotene, plus liver and dairy products.
Vitamin C	May protect against certain types of cancer, such as cancer of the oesophagus and stomach.	Good sources include broccoli, cauliflower, green peppers, strawberries and citrus fruits.
Vitamin E	May help protect against cancers of the oesophagus and stomach.	Found in wholegrain cereals and unsaturated vegetable oils.
Selenium	May help protect against cancers of the oesophagus and stomach.	Good sources include fish, brazil nuts and most wholegrains.

5

PREVENTING INFECTIONS

The immune system, like all other body systems, needs the right fuel if it is to function efficiently. If the body does not receive the right nutrients one of the earliest consequences is an increased susceptibility to infections of all kinds, in particular, viral infections such as colds and flu. Viruses such as colds and flu normally start with mild symptoms such as a congested feeling in the nose and throat and slight fever. At this stage the body is beginning to resist the infection and taking certain courses of action may actually help the body fight the infection and stop the illness developing any further.

WHO IS AT RISK

All of us are at some risk from infection every day of our lives. However, some groups need to take particular care to keep their immune system working at its best. You may have an increased risk of infection if any of the following apply in your case:

■ You are recovering from any kind of illness.

■ You work in a place where you are likely to be exposed to infection – for example, a hospital or school.

■ You are taking medication that may suppress the immune system, such as corticosteroids or anticancer drugs.

■ You are elderly or in generally poor health.

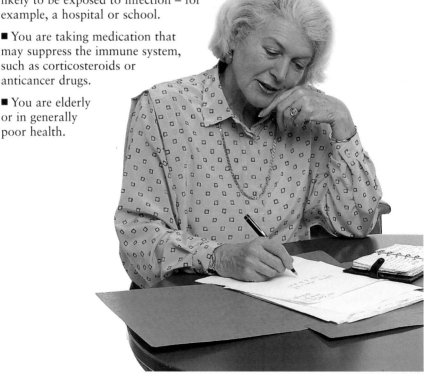

5

KEY NUTRIENTS

The key nutrients for immune health are vitamin C, beta-carotene and the mineral zinc. Therefore if you think you are at risk from infection you need to be sure to include adequate amounts of these nutrients in your diet.

■ **Vitamin C** Eat plenty of fruit; citrus fruits, bananas and kiwi fruits are all excellent sources. Green leafy vegetables are also rich in vitamin C. Taking large doses of vitamin C when symptoms of infection first become apparent may prevent the illness from progressing, and will usually reduce its duration or severity. The normal dose is 1 g of vitamin C every 1–2 hours until the symptoms have disappeared.

■ **Beta-carotene** This is found in high concentrations in yellow and orange fruit and vegetables such as apricots, carrots, and red and yellow peppers. Make sure you include these in your diet.

■ **Zinc** Seafood, fish and wholegrains are good sources of zinc.

FOOD FACTORS THAT REDUCE RESISTANCE

Apart from making sure your diet includes the nutrients that positively enhance your body's ability to fight off infection, it is also important to exclude those factors related to diet that can inhibit the healthy functioning of the immune system or make the symptoms of infection worse.

■ **Avoid heavy meals** When the body has to cope with large meals, its ability to combat infection is reduced. To optimize your infection-fighting capabilities, avoid large meals, in particular those that contain large amounts of "heavy" or fatty foods such as meat and dairy products.

■ **Reduce sugar intake** As the level of sugar in the bloodstream rises, the efficiency of the immune system is reduced. To give your body the best chance of resisting infection it therefore makes sense to reduce your intake of sugar, sweet drinks and sugar-containing foods, such as biscuits and cakes.

■ **Avoid mucus-forming foods** If you have or are developing a cold, it may be helpful to cut down on foods that encourage the formation of mucus. The most important foods to avoid are cow's milk and cow's milk products such as cheese.

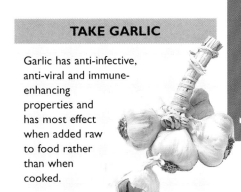

TAKE GARLIC

Garlic has anti-infective, anti-viral and immune-enhancing properties and has most effect when added raw to food rather than when cooked.

5

RHEUMATOID ARTHRITIS

R heumatoid arthritis is what is known as an "auto-immune" disease – the body's immune system mounts an immune response against its own tissues, causing inflammation and diseased tissue. In the case of rheumatoid arthritis, the part of the body affected is the tissue that lines the joint known as the synovium. It usually starts in early adulthood or middle age but can sometimes start in childhood. Rheumatoid arthritis affects 2–3 per cent of the population and about 75 per cent of sufferers are women. The cause of rheumatoid arthritis is not known, but there is some evidence that it can be triggered by food.

KEY SYMPTOMS

Rheumatoid arthritis is characterized by inflammation in the joints of the fingers, toes, wrists or other joints of the body. The affected joints become swollen and stiff and may become deformed in the long term. People with the condition are also likely to feel generally unwell. The disease usually comes in waves, with painful periods being interspersed with times where sufferers are relatively symptom-free.

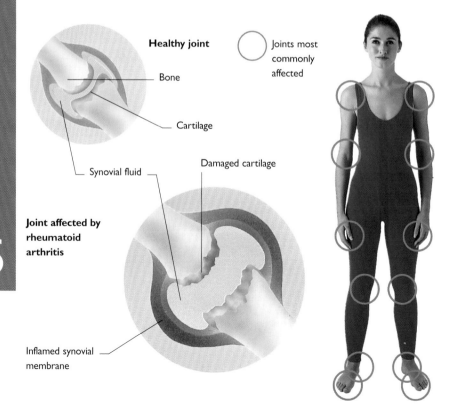

Healthy joint

Bone

Cartilage

Synovial fluid

Joints most commonly affected

Damaged cartilage

Joint affected by rheumatoid arthritis

Inflamed synovial membrane

5

FOODS AND RHEUMATOID ARTHRITIS

■ **Avoid foods that tend to cause inflammation.** There are some foods that we eat on a day-to-day basis that seem to promote the processes that cause inflammation in the body, such as red meat, sugar and coffee. Cutting back on these foods or eliminating them altogether may help to reduce the symptoms of rheumatoid arthritis.

■ **Avoid foods to which you may be sensitive.** In some individuals, the immune system activity that causes rheumatoid arthritis seems to be triggered by certain foods. It is thought that partially digested food leaks through the intestinal wall into the bloodstream, going on to trigger the immune cells to react. Common culprits in these reactions include wheat, corn, dairy products and citrus fruits. A significant number of rheumatoid arthritis sufferers find that identifying and eliminating problem foods from the diet can lead to significant improvement in their symptoms.

NATURAL ANTI-INFLAMMATORY FOODS

While some foods tend to encourage inflammation in the body, others have the reverse effect. Healthy fats, also known as essential fatty acids, in the diet are metabolized in the body into substances that have natural anti-inflammatory properties. Foods that are rich in these healthy fats include oily fish such as mackerel, salmon and trout, olive oil and pumpkin, sunflower and sesame seeds, and increased amounts of these foods are recommended.

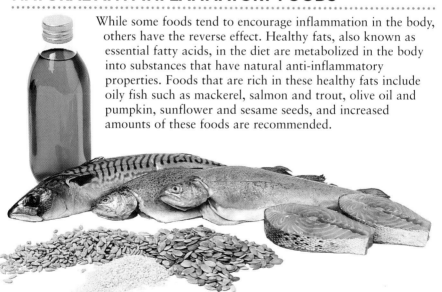

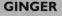

GINGER

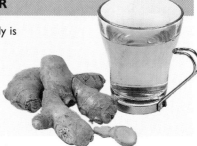

A food that helps reduce inflammation naturally is ginger. It can be added to stir-fries and other dishes, or it may be taken as an infusion or "tea". This is made by steeping some freshly sliced or grated root ginger in hot water.

5

IMMUNE-BOOSTING MEALS

The following menu plans provide ideas for meals that may help to keep the immune system strong and healthy. The meals are based on foods that are rich in the immune-boosting and cancer-preventing nutrients such as vitamins C and E and the minerals zinc and selenium. They are also low in the food elements that may tend to weaken the immune system or help promote cancer such as sugar and fat.

BREAKFASTS FOR IMMUNE HEALTH

Depending on how hungry you are in the morning and how physically strenuous the day ahead, choose one or more items from these suggestions.

- Low-sugar, oat-based muesli with skimmed milk or soya milk and fruit topping.

- Fresh fruit.

- Blended fruit smoothie made with kiwi fruit and bananas, low-fat yoghurt and ice.

- Dried fruit compote with added fresh citrus fruit.

- Fresh or grilled grapefruit, sprinkled with cinnamon, if liked.

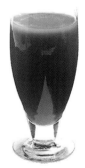

- Porridge made with skimmed milk and topped with dried or fresh fruit.

- Unsweetened wholewheat-based cereal with added dried or fresh fruit plus skimmed milk or soya milk.

- Freshly squeezed orange juice followed by live yoghurt with fruit.

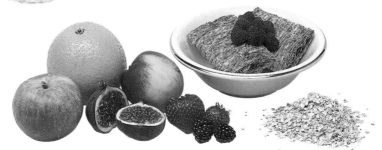

5

LUNCHES FOR IMMUNE HEALTH

The key to immune health is to maintain your intake of fresh fruit and vegetables. Even if you have only time for a sandwich, you can still look after your immune system by opting for wholegrain bread with a salad-based filling. Choose fresh fruit for dessert.

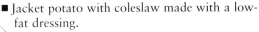

■ Stuffed peppers and brown rice.

■ Avocado salad sandwich on wholegrain bread.

■ Fresh vegetable soup with wholegrain bread or rye crackers.

■ Avocado dip with sticks of raw vegetables.

■ Cracked wheat salad (such as tabbouleh) topped with toasted seeds (sesame, sunflower or pumpkin).

■ Vegetable or chick pea burger or rissole with wholemeal bread (wholemeal Greek pitta bread is ideal) and a green salad tossed in extra virgin olive oil and lemon juice.

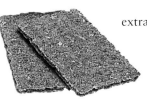

■ Jacket potato with coleslaw made with a low-fat dressing.

■ Sardine, tuna or salmon pâté with wholemeal crackers or crispbread and green salad.

■ Avocado and prawn or crab salad with a low-fat yoghurt dressing.

■ Grilled peppers and courgettes with extra virgin olive oil and brown rice.

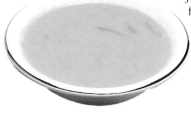

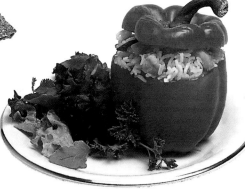

5

EVENING MEALS FOR IMMUNE HEALTH

Immune-boosting nutrients are often destroyed by lengthy cooking, so be sure to include raw or lightly cooked vegetables in your evening meal. Finish the meal with a fruit-based dessert of your choice.

■ White fish, such as plaice, with watercress sauce, steamed vegetables and baked or boiled potatoes.

■ Seafood and vegetable stir-fry served with egg noodles.

■ Grilled mackerel or herring with apple sauce, boiled potatoes and steamed vegetables.

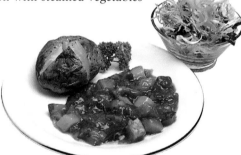

■ Salmon baked with lemon and dill served with steamed vegetables or salad.

■ Stuffed aubergine, mushrooms or marrow served with wholegrain bread and salad.

■ Wholewheat pasta with a sauce made from spinach, pinenuts, extra virgin olive oil and garlic.

■ Liver sautéed in extra virgin olive oil with steamed vegetables and boiled potatoes.

■ Chicken, vegetable or fish risotto made with brown rice.

■ Vegetable goulash with baked potato and side salad.

■ Bean casserole with steamed vegetables.

DESSERT SUGGESTIONS

■ Fruit purée with yoghurt.

■ Low-fat fromage frais with fresh fruit salad.

■ Citrus fruit salad.

■ Poached pears with blackcurrant or raspberry coulis, sweetened with honey.

■ Banana or mango frozen yoghurt dessert (mashed fruit mixed with natural yoghurt and whipped egg whites frozen until solid).

■ Fruit jelly made with unsweeted fruit juice and fresh fruit pieces.

5

SHOPPING AND COOKING

The importance of food in ensuring good health and combating illness cannot be exaggerated. However, converting theoretical knowledge into healthy dietary changes means knowing how to shop for and prepare food for optimum health. As well as choosing healthy main ingredients, you will need to prepare them using a minimum of unhealthy ones mixed with them, such as fat, salt and sugar. However, by following a few simple rules, you will be able to plan and prepare delicious, healthy meals for you and your family.

SHOPPING FOR FOOD

Many people regard the weekly food shopping trip to the supermarket as a chore to be completed as fast as possible. However, the selection of food in the shop is your first step to healthy eating and should be given careful thought and consideration. The following shopping tips should help you get the most out of your trips to the local food store.

AVOID SHOPPING ON AN EMPTY STOMACH

Food stores and supermarkets are full of tempting but generally unhealthy foods such as cakes, biscuits and confectionery. Resisting these foods is almost impossible when we are hungry and the craving for instant energy is high, so shopping on an empty stomach almost inevitably leads to us making unhealthy food choices. Eating before you shop will help ensure you choose your food in a controlled, health-conscious manner.

CHOOSING FRUIT AND VEGETABLES

■ Choose fresh fruit and vegetables unless convenience is an overwhelming priority. These generally contain more nutrients than their frozen or canned versions. Canned vegetables usually contain significant amounts of salt and sugar which may have an adverse effect on health in the long term.

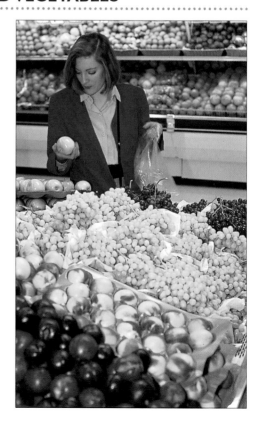

■ When choosing fresh vegetables, go for smaller, younger produce as these are usually tastier and contain higher concentrations of nutrients than larger, older specimens. Generally, the darker the vegetable, the more nutritious it is – so opt for deep orange carrots and dark green leafy vegetables.

■ Pick up fruit and vegetables and inspect them for bruising and discoloration. Feel produce to assess freshness and ripeness.

6

CHOOSING BREAD, PASTA AND RICE

When choosing cereals such as bread, rice and pasta, the most important thing is to buy them in their least refined form. Wholemeal bread, wholewheat pasta and brown rice are to be preferred to their refined versions. Make sure the bread you buy is labelled 100 per cent wholegrain. Many brown breads contain a substantial proportion of white flour. Nutritionally, there is not much to choose between fresh and dried pasta. Fresh pasta is quicker to cook but is also more expensive.

CHOOSING MEAT, POULTRY AND FISH

■ The watchword to bear in mind when choosing meat, poultry and fish is fat. The healthiest option is fish. Oily fish such as mackerel, salmon and trout contain fats that have an important role to play in health, particularly in the prevention of heart disease. Avoid prepared fish products that are covered in batter or breadcrumbs as these are likely to contain more unhealthy fat than fresh fish.

■ Poultry is relatively low in fat as long as the skin is discarded before cooking. If you do buy red meat, choose lean cuts which have had the fat already trimmed. Venison is one red meat that is actually relatively low in fat.

CHOOSING DAIRY PRODUCTS

■ Skimmed milk is the most healthy form of milk as it contains virtually no fat. Semi-skimmed milk also makes a healthy alternative to full-fat milk with approximately half the fat content.

■ Cheeses are either ripened (such as cheddar, gruyère, brie and parmesan) or unripened (such as cottage, cream, mozzarella, ricotta). Unripened cheeses are preferable as they generally contain less fat and cholesterol compared with the ripened cheeses.

■ Live, natural, unsweetened yoghurt is the healthiest form of yoghurt. Fruit yoghurts tend to contain large amounts of sugar or artificial sweeteners such as aspartame, and may also have added thickening agents.

6

WHERE TO SHOP

It is generally more convenient to shop in stores which offer a variety of foods rather than speciality shops such as butchers or bakers. However, you may find that specialist shops offer a better selection of free-range or organic products. While certain food items are available only at health food stores, many can also be found in supermarkets. Each kind of shop has its advantages and disadvantages.

SUPERMARKET OR HEALTH FOOD STORE?

Overall choice	Supermarkets tend to stock a wider variety of items, enabling you to complete your shopping in one store.	Health food stores are likely to have a better range of wholegrain and organic products, as well as nuts and seeds.
Dairy produce	Supermarkets generally have a wide selection of standard dairy items.	Health food stores are more likely to stock non-cow's milk produce such as goat's and sheep's milk and cheese, as well as soya products.
Organic produce	Supermarkets tend to stock only a limited amount of organic produce.	Health food stores generally provide a wide variety of organic food items.
Fruit and vegetables	With their larger shelf space and rapid turnover, supermarkets are likely to offer more choice and the produce is likely to be fresher.	Health food stores may stock organic produce that is often unavailable in supermarkets.
Non-wheat alternatives	Supermarkets may have a limited choice of non-wheat alternatives to standard products such as pasta and flour.	Health food stores are often the best place to find corn- or rice-based pasta, non-wheat flours and other grains such as millet.

6

SUPERMARKET OR HEALTH FOOD STORE?

Meat and fish	Supermarkets normally offer a wide variety of meat and fish items, both frozen and fresh.	It is rare for these products to be stocked by health food stores and, if they do, the range is generally very limited.
Beans and pulses	Supermarkets generally stock standard, non-organic varieties.	Health food stores normally offer a wide variety of beans and pulses, many of which may be found in organic form.
Breakfast cereals	Supermarkets usually offer a very wide variety of breakfast cereals, but these are predominantly of the sugar- and salt-laden variety.	Cereals found in health food stores are likely to be lower in sugar. Non-wheat breakfast cereals are also more likely to be stocked.
Low-sugar items	Supermarkets may offer some low-sugar products but these may be high in artificial alternatives.	In a health food store you will be more likely to find low-sugar products that contain healthier alternatives to normal sugar, such as fruit juice or honey.
Wholegrain items	Some wholegrain items such as brown rice are easy to find in supermarkets, but choice may be limited.	Certain items such as 100 per cent wholegrain wheat or rye bread is usually more easily found in a health food store.

FINDING ADVICE

If you want to find healthy alternatives to commonly eaten foods, or want information about the nutritional merit of the food you are buying, you are much more likely to get helpful advice in a health food store than a supermarket.

6

LOW-FAT COOKING

One of the fundamentals of any healthy eating plan must be to cut down on the amount of fat consumed in the diet. Apart from making low-fat food choices, the other major area in which we reduce fat intake is in food preparation. This section looks at how food may be prepared and cooked with a view to reducing fat consumption.

LOW-FAT COOKING METHODS

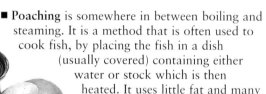

Many cooking methods do not require the addition of fat. The most healthy of all cooking methods is probably steaming.

■ **Steaming** is fast, fat-free and causes minimal nutrient loss. It is the most suitable method of cooking for fish and vegetables.

■ **Boiling** is an alternative to steaming though the nutrient losses tend to be greater.

■ **Poaching** is somewhere in between boiling and steaming. It is a method that is often used to cook fish, by placing the fish in a dish (usually covered) containing either water or stock which is then heated. It uses little fat and many nutrients are preserved.

■ **No-fat roasting or baking** can be used to cook joints of meat and poultry. No oil or fat should be added before or during the cooking process and the meat should be put on a rack so that the fat in the meat has the opportunity to drain properly from the meat.

■ **Grilling** is a low-fat method of cooking for thinner cuts of meat, poultry, fish and certain vegetables such as tomatoes and peppers. Char-grilled food should be avoided because there is some association between this and the risk of certain cancers.

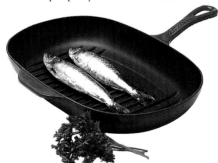

AVOID SHALLOW AND DEEP-FRIED FOOD

Any sort of frying adds significant quantities of fat to food and is therefore best avoided. Not only does the fat coat the outside of the food, it is also absorbed into the food. What is more, heating oil to the high temperature required for frying can change the nature of the oil itself, too, making it more harmful to the body. Stir-frying is the least harmful of the frying methods in that it uses only a small amount of oil.

USE NON-STICK KITCHEN UTENSILS

If you need to fry food – for example, when stir-frying – use a non-stick frying pan or saucepan to cut down on the amount of oil or fat used. Remove the food from the pan as soon as it is cooked.

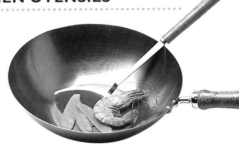

REMOVE SKIN AND EXCESS FAT

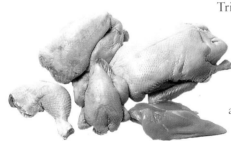

Trim the fat from meat and remove the skin from poultry before cooking. Removing as much fat as possible before cooking dishes such as casseroles and stews helps to ensure that as little fat as possible ends up on the plate. After cooking, chill meat stews and soups to allow the fat to rise to the top and solidify. Spoon off the fat and discard before re-heating and serving.

USE LOW-FAT DAIRY PRODUCTS IN RECIPES

Full-fat milk can simply be replaced with skimmed or semi-skimmed versions in cooking. Cream can be mixed half and half with low-fat natural yoghurt. It is possible to use a low-fat cheese instead of the full-fat variety in most recipes. Even when some form of fat such as butter is called for, the quantity of fat can usually be reduced by a third without affecting texture or taste.

6

FLAVOURING FOOD

Reducing salt and sugar consumption is important if you are to have a healthy diet. You may be pleasantly surprised at the range of subtle flavours that can be savoured when you cut down on the culinary "sledgehammers" of salt and sugar and try some of the following healthy alternatives.

ALTERNATIVES TO SALT

There is good evidence that, because of its effect on blood pressure, salt can increase the risk of major conditions such as heart disease and stroke. However, there are several alternatives to regular table salt.

Unrefined sea salt

Unrefined sea salt is rich in a wide range of minerals and trace minerals which may help to offset the potentially harmful effects of regular salt. It can be found in good health food stores. However, like ordinary salt, it should be used sparingly.

High-potassium, low-sodium salt

Salt based on potassium chloride rather than sodium chloride is now widely available and almost certainly offers significant health benefits over table salt which is made almost entirely from sodium chloride. Some studies also indicate that potassium can help lower blood pressure.

Ground dried vegetables or herbs

There are some salt substitutes based on ground dried vegetables and herbs or dried herbs alone. These can be used as natural flavour enhancers and can reduce or even eliminate the need for regular salt in a recipe.

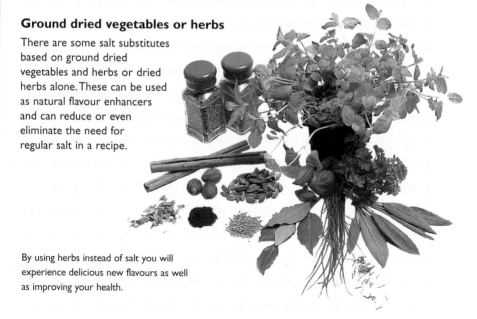

By using herbs instead of salt you will experience delicious new flavours as well as improving your health.

6

ALTERNATIVES TO SUGAR

Sugar, whether white or brown, is a highly refined foodstuff with almost no nutritional value. The following list provides some alternatives to sugar.

Honey

Raw (unrefined) honey releases sugar more slowly into the bloodstream than sugar and may also contain a small amount of vitamins and minerals.

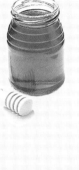

Blackstrap molasses

A good alternative to sugar in cakes and biscuits, blackstrap molasses are a significant source of vitamins B_1, B_2 and B_3 and iron, calcium and potassium.

Maple syrup

This is generally less sweet and more mineral rich than sugar. Look for a product that is 100 per cent maple syrup as many commercially available products are made of water, sugar and maple syrup flavouring.

Fruit purée or concentrate

These products, often based on pineapple, pear, grape or other fruit, retain some of their original nutrients, making them excellent for addition to biscuits and cakes or as a topping for breakfast cereal. You can buy them in health food stores or make them by blending chopped fresh fruit with a small amount of fruit juice.

Dates, raisins and other dried fruit

These can be added to cakes, biscuits and other foods for natural sweetness.

Fresh fruit

Fruit is the ideal natural sweetener for breakfast cereal or plain yoghurt.

Malt syrup

Malt syrup made from barley or rice contains some of the nutrients from the original grains including vitamins K, B, A and C and the mineral calcium. You can buy it from health food stores.

Liquorice root

This can give a pleasantly sweet taste to herbal tea.

Stevia

Stevia is a sweet substance extracted from a South American plant. It can be used in baking or beverages. A little of this extract goes a very long way.

6

EATING DAY-BY-DAY

The pages outline healthy menus for two weeks. The ingredients for the menus have been chosen to ensure that the overall nutritional content of each meal is low in fat and sugar, while being high in fibre and health-giving nutrients. The meal suggestions are not to be adhered to slavishly. It is possible to adapt menus to suit you or your family's tastes without affecting their overall nutritional value.

DAY ONE

Breakfast
Porridge made with skimmed milk with fresh or dried fruit.

Lunch
Tuna salad sandwich made with 100 per cent wholegrain wheat or rye bread. Fresh fruit.

Evening meal
Pasta with tomato-based sauce and salad dressed with extra virgin olive oil and lemon juice. Fresh fruit.

DAY TWO

Breakfast
Low-sugar or no-sugar breakfast cereal with skimmed milk and added fruit and seeds (sesame, sunflower or pumpkin).

Lunch
Vegetable soup, wholegrain bread or rye crackers. Fresh fruit.

Evening meal
Chicken satay and raw vegetable sticks with yoghurt-based or thin peanut sauce and salad. Fresh fruit.

DAY THREE

Breakfast
Grapefruit followed by a boiled or poached egg with wholegrain toast.

Lunch
Avocado salad sandwich made with 100 per cent wholegrain bread. Fresh fruit.

Evening meal
Stir-fried prawns and vegetables with noodles. Fresh fruit.

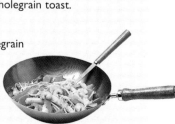

DAY FOUR

Breakfast
Fresh fruit salad with low-fat natural yoghurt.

Lunch
Oatmeal-coated grilled mackerel or herring with steamed vegetables or salad.
Fresh fruit.

Evening meal
Grilled skinless chicken (marinated, if desired, in extra virgin olive oil, lemon juice, garlic and herbs) with boiled potatoes and steamed vegetables. Unsweetened fruit crumble, with oat or muesli topping.

DAY FIVE

Breakfast
Unsweetened muesli with skimmed milk and fresh fruit or fruit purée.

Lunch
Fresh vegetable soup with 100 per cent wholegrain bread or rye crackers. Fresh fruit.

Evening meal
Grilled or poached trout or salmon with steamed vegetables. Fruit purée served with low-fat yoghurt or fromage frais.

DAY SIX

Breakfast
100 per cent wholegrain wheat or rye toast with no-sugar-added jam, plus a piece of fruit.

Lunch
Brown rice salad containing grilled chicken, peppers, carrot, tomato and chick peas, dressed with extra virgin olive oil and balsamic vinegar.
Fresh fruit.

Evening meal
Vegetable and bean casserole with steamed vegetables. Poached pears with blackcurrant or raspberry coulis sweetened with honey.

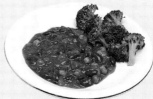

6

DAY SEVEN

Breakfast
Low-sugar, oat-based muesli with skimmed milk or soya milk and fruit topping.

Lunch
Avocado dip with raw vegetable sticks. Fresh fruit.

Evening meal
Chicken casserole with brown rice and steamed green vegetables. Citrus fruit salad.

DAY EIGHT

Breakfast
Unsweetened breakfast cereal made with skimmed milk and topped with some fresh fruit or fruit purée.

Lunch
Chicken salad sandwich made with 100 per cent wholegrain bread. Fresh fruit.

Evening meal
Baked fish with breadcrumb topping, steamed vegetables and baked potato. Fresh fruit or low-fat yoghurt.

DAY NINE

Breakfast
Dried fruit compote with fresh orange segments, low-fat natural yoghurt.

Lunch
Fish pâté on wholegrain bread or crackers, side salad. Fresh fruit.

Evening meal
Lean meat steak (such as venison) served with boiled potatoes and steamed vegetables. Fresh fruit.

DAY TEN

Breakfast
Oat porridge made with skimmed milk topped with banana.

Lunch
Jacket potato topped with tuna and sweetcorn with green salad. Fresh fruit.

Evening meal
Ratatouille with brown rice. Fresh fruit.

6

DAY ELEVEN

Breakfast
Blended kiwi fruit and banana smoothie, made with low-fat yoghurt and ice.

Lunch
Fish cakes and salad. Fresh fruit.

Evening meal
Sautéed liver with salad or steamed vegetables and new potatoes. Fresh fruit salad with low-fat fromage frais.

DAY TWELVE

Breakfast
Oat or bran muffin. Fresh fruit.

Lunch
Jacket potato with plain or flavoured cottage cheese, or tuna and sweetcorn with reduced fat crème fraîche. Fresh fruit.

Evening meal
Seafood and vegetable stir-fry with egg noodles and salad. Fresh fruit topped with natural yoghurt and sprinkled with brown sugar and grilled until caramelized.

DAY THIRTEEN

Breakfast
Cottage cheese and wholegrain toast. Fresh fruit.

Lunch
Sardines on wholegrain toast with grilled tomatoes. Fresh fruit.

Evening meal
Lentil or bean casserole, steamed vegetables. Fresh fruit or low-fat yoghurt.

DAY FOURTEEN

Breakfast
Blended fruit smoothie containing fresh fruit, low-fat yoghurt, oat germ, and ice with a little fruit purée, honey or maple syrup.

Lunch
Smoked mackerel salad with extra virgin olive oil and lemon juice. Fresh fruit.

Evening meal
Vegetable goulash with baked potato and side salad dressed with extra virgin olive oil. Banana or mango frozen yoghurt dessert (mashed fruit mixed with natural yoghurt and whipped egg whites frozen until solid).

6

INDEX

A
acid reflux 50
ageing, slowing 22
anti-oxidants
  and cancer 87
  and free radicals 23
  and the heart 37
artificial sweeteners 33
auto-immune diseases 83

B
beta-carotene 23
  and cancer 91
  and immune system 85
blood sugar 12
  and weight 74
  low 13
  sustaining 14
body fat percentage (BFP) 66
body mass index (BMI) 62
bones, healthy 20

C
caffeine 26
  in diet drinks 77
calcium 17
  and bone growth 20
cancer 86
  and alcohol 89
  and diet 88
  anti-cancer foods 90
candida 55
carbohydrate 11
cholesterol 29
  reducing 31
constipation 54

D
diabetes mellitus 12
diet drinks 77

dieting pitfalls 64
digestion 46

E
energy 8
  and alcohol 26
  foods for 24
  nutrients for 16
  sappers 26
  stores 10
exercise 18
  and bone health 21
  and constipation 55

F
fat 11
  and cancer 88
  and the heart 29
  male/female 68
fatigue 74
  and low energy 12
fats 30
  healthy 37
fibre
  and cancer 90
  and digestion 54
  and IBS 58
flavouring food 106
fluid intake
  and constipation 55
  and exercise 19
food combining 52
food intolerance 70
  and IBS 57
  and immune response 84
  signs/symptoms of 72
food myths 76
free radicals
  and ageing 22
  and anti-oxidants 36
  and cancer 88

G, H, I
glycaemic index 75
  foods 15
glycogen 10
  stores 18

gout 20
heart
  alcohol and the 40
  cooking for the 38
  disease 28
  meals for the 42
heartburn 50
hiatus hernia 50
high blood pressure 34
hypoglycaemia 13
immune response
  and weight gain 70
  food sensitivity and 84
immune system 82
  diet and 84
  meals for 96
  nutrients for 93
  problems with 82
indigestion 49
infections, preventing 92
insulin 12
irritable bowel syndrome (IBS) 56
  foods to relieve 58

L, M
lipoproteins (LDL, HDL) 29
low-fat
  cooking 104
  foods 76
magnesium 17
  and bone growth 20
meal size 85
Mediterranean diet 30
menopause 23
menus, day-by-day 108

O, P, Q
obesity 62
  and cancer 90
oestrogen 23
osteoporosis 21
overweight 62
potassium 17
protein 11
rheumatoid arthritis 94

S, T
salt 34
  alternatives to 106
selenium 23
  and cancer 91
shopping for food 100
  where to shop 102
slimming foods 77
sugar 32
  alternatives to 107
  and immune health 85
sugary foods and drinks 26
tiredness 13
trans fats (TFAs) 88
triglycerides 32

U, V
ulcers 51
vitamins
  A 23
  B_1 16
  B_2 16
  B_3 16
  B_5 16
  B_{12} 16
  C 23
  E 23

W, Y, Z
water see fluid intake
weight 62
  control plan 79
  loss, lasting 78
weight-cycling 65
yeast organisms 57
zinc 85

ACKNOWLEDGMENTS
The author and the publishers gratefully acknowledge the invaluable contributions made by Laura Wickenden who took all the photographs in this book except:
p. 13 T.C. Mettier/Zefa; p. 20 (top right) Zefa; p. 21 (bottom) Prof. P. Motta/Science Photo Library; p. 30 (top) Romilly Lockyer/Image Bank; p. 55 (bottom) Nancy Brown/Image Bank; p. 71 Chris Harvey/Tony Stone; p. 73 BSIP Boucharlat/Science Phot Library; p. 87 G. Palmer/Zefa; p. 89 (centre) Grimberg/Image Bank; p. 92 Zefa; p. 100 Don and Pat Valenti/Tony Stone.
The illustrations were produced by Chris Forsey and Janos Marffy. Additional charts and diagrams by Nick Buzzard.